THE
SELF-HELP REFLEXOLOGY HANDBOOK

THE SELF-HELP
Reflexology
Handbook

**Easy routines for hands and feet
to enhance health and vitality**

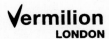
Vermilion
LONDON

First published 1997

9 10 8

First published in the United Kingdom by Vermilion
An imprint of Ebury Press
The Random House Group Ltd
Random House
20 Vauxhall Bridge Road
London SW1V 2SA

The Random House Group Limited Reg. No. 954009
www.randomhouse.co.uk

A CIP catalogue record for this book is available from the British Library

ISBN 9780091815370

Illustrations by Emma Dodd except for
James Horan's maps illustrated by Heather Hacking

Penguin Random House is committed to a sustainable future for our business, our readers and our planet. This book is made from Forest Stewardship Council® certified paper.

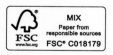

Printed and bound in Great Britain by Clays Ltd, St Ives plc

Please note that any information offered in this book is not intended to replace medical advice from a doctor, consultant or any medical health advisor.
Please consult your doctor before receiving or practising any of the self-help reflexology techniques, routines or workouts in this book.

CONTENTS

Acknowledgements

Thank you to Lillian and William Ducie and to all my friends for their love and encouragement along the way.

FOREWORD

We have a natural ability to heal ourselves. In the dawn of mankind, we used to walk around barefoot and the stones underfoot massaged our feet, but we have come a long way since then – such things as cement pavements, shoes, the car and supermarkets have made our lives so much easier, but have taken us away from things natural. However nature is adaptable and just as we can have a good workout to compensate for a day spent inactive at a desk, so too we can use self-help techniques to compensate for the forced and sometimes inappropriate changes to our lifestyle.

This book is dedicated to self-help and self-healing through a very simple, yet very powerful therapy called reflexology. It can help you find optimum health and help prevent illness. The need is great. The World Health Organisation has a vision – good health for all by the year 2000 – yet as the millennium fast draws to a close, alarming statistics show that although people are generally living longer, they are not necessarily living in optimum health with diseases such as cancer, heart disease, rheumatism, arthritis, back problems and asthma on the increase.

Sonia Ducie encourages us to take a look at that vastly underrated part of our anatomy – the feet. We totally underestimate the importance of the feet. They get you to where you need to be to do your great work. They say that by the time we are 70 we will have walked the equivalent of three times around the world!

Have you ever watched children play on a beach? They rush around irrespective of the pebbles underfoot, but as we get older, we may wince as we gingerly pick our way across, trying to avoid them. The reason is simple. Through the pollutants in the air we breathe, the food we eat and the liquid we drink, any negative thinking, lack of exercise, uncontrolled stress and poor lifestyle generally, toxins build up throughout the nerve pathways of our body, which end up in our hands and feet. This causes an imbalance to the body; it creates factors which weaken our immune systems and hence can lead us from dis-ease to illness. It basically creates sore feet. An example of this is coming home after a long day, feeling dreadful. You may say something like, 'Oh, my feet are killing me,' then kick off your shoes and even rub your feet.

This book helps you to take charge of your own health and assist the body in its own healing. Additionally, it will help you to help those in your own circle – your family and friends. It could even inspire you to take up reflexology as a profession. Keep this book by your side. It could change your life!

– Mo Usher, MAR, MGCP

Mo Usher is honorary life member and former President of the Association of Reflexologists and was their Chairman for six years. She has served as President of the International Council of Reflexologists and was honoured for her work as one of the 'Best of British Women' in 1993.

How to Use This Book

The Self-Help Reflexology Handbook offers you a chance to learn some simple reflexology techniques which can help you relax and stay healthy. It inspires and motivates you to include regular reflexology in your life, along with exercise, fresh air, a healthy diet, etc., to help keep you balanced, happy and glowing with confidence. When you are healthy and happy you are able to put more into life, and because reflexology helps increase your creativity, it can even help to make you more efficient! By being a happier, more caring person you will naturally make others around you happier, too.

Practising reflexology brings self-awareness about how your body works and what it needs, and teaches you to take responsibility for yourself. It's your body, after all – and when you look after it with love, care and attention, it will look after you.

This isn't a medical book that tells you how to diagnose your symptoms and practising the self-help techniques isn't going to cure you of all ills – but it can help. The book has been designed so you can obtain the maximum benefits from your reflexology routines and workouts:

INTRODUCTION
Here you will find a review of the history of reflexology and how it is used today, to give you a background on the subject. Also, *this section* contains general information about reflexology, what it can and can't do, and notes on what to expect from the self-help approach.

HEALING, THE AURA AND THE CHAKRAS
All life is made up of energy, or ch'i, as it is sometimes known. The human aura is the electromagnetic energy field that surrounds you, while chakras are seven vortices of moving energy, running at intervals along your spine, which energize the organs of your body.

THE SYSTEMS OF THE BODY
If you don't remember much of your school biology, then read this short synopsis to get a little understanding of how your body functions.

WARMING UP
Warming up is an important part of your routine and this section also gives you tips on how to get the most out of your routines, whether in the office, travelling or at home.

GENERAL RELAXATION TECHNIQUES
This is the most important part of the book because it explains the basic reflexology movement – the caterpillar movement – and other relaxation techniques which need to be practised before and after any of the self-help routines or workouts.

HOW WILL REFLEXOLOGY MAKE ME FEEL?
You may also like to read about typical reactions to reflexology in this section.

DOS AND DON'TS CHECKLIST
Before practising any of the self-help techniques in Part III (Common Health Complaints), have a general check-up

with your doctor, who has your full medical history and knows about your health. This checklist highlights some of the many points you may like to discuss together.

SELF-HELP FOR ENERGY AND VITALITY
INTRODUCTION AND WORKOUTS
Everyone wants to make the most of life and reflexology can help give you the energy and vitality do just that. Also, loving yourself, valuing yourself and feeling good about who you are will help make you radiate with confidence and look beautiful!

SELF-HELP FOR HEALTH
Introduction and Common Complaints Here is a list of common complaints which may be experienced in daily life and self-help routines to help you manage them.

VISITING A PROFESSIONAL THERAPIST
At some point, either before you start working on your own self-help routines or after a while, you may like to visit a professional reflexologist for a treatment. This may be out of curiosity, for pampering and general relaxation, or because you are ill. This chapter covers everything from what to wear to choosing your reflexologist and how to find out the cost of a treatment.

PROFESSIONAL ASSOCIATIONS/
READING LIST
At the back of the book is a contact list of fully trained reflexologists and a list of a few of the many exciting reflexology books available today.

JIM HORAN'S HAND AND FEET CHARTS
Each workout or self-help routine in this book has a number for each reflex point and they are illustrated here. If your routine is shown using hand reflexology and you wish to use foot reflexology instead, then simply look up those numbers on these charts. They will also give you an idea of your whole body and how it works.

Before you practise any of the self-help techniques in this book it is essential that you read the 'Dos and Don'ts Checklist' (page 34), then 'Warming Up' (page 35) and 'How Will It Make Me Feel' (page 32) to help you understand the process. Always remember to practise the general relaxation techniques for a few minutes before and after any of your routines or workouts, as reflexology works on the whole body.

This book is your friend – it's here to help you to get the most out of your life and your health. So have fun, relax and enjoy the journey ahead.

INTRODUCTION

What Is Reflexology?

Reflexology is a wonderful, natural and simple way of helping your body to heal itself. It is often referred to as a holistic therapy, meaning 'whole', because it works on your whole mind, body and spirit, rather than focusing on your symptoms. When you are sick, reflexology is nurturing, healing, relaxing and invigorating, and when you are healthy its healing touch helps to make you feel good in yourself, positive and happy. Regular reflexology can help prevent certain reoccurrences of illness and help maintain your health. It is practised by professional therapists all over the world, in health centres, hospitals, at home and even in the workplace. Everyone can benefit from it, from young children to the elderly, in sickness and in health, for fun and for pleasure, for mind, body and spirit.

Mapped out on your feet and hands are 'reflex points' which correspond to every organ and part of your body. When you are ill or stressed these points become sensitive and sore to touch, as toxins build up. These toxins cause blockages in your body which prevent your energies from flowing freely. Reflexologists can feel toxins or crystal deposits just underneath the skin. By working over the areas of congestion, the blockages are released, which helps to bring your body back into balance and harmony.

Reflexology is sometimes referred to as 'zone therapy', because every one of your reflex points lies within a certain zone or meridian. Your body is divided into 10 equal zones; when you draw a line vertically down the middle of your body there are exactly five zones running down either side. These zones are also sometimes referred to as 'energy pathways' or 'nerve pathways'. Every part of your body is connected to the rest and so a blockage of energy in one zone will affect the whole. Therefore it is important to look after your whole self, from your head to your toes, through a healthy diet, exercise, relaxation and plenty of sleep, and to find a balance in work and play.

Reflexology encourages you to breathe, to relax and to let go of stress. Stress has been suggested as the cause of a great many illnesses; some people say as many as 80 per cent. A little stress is necessary – it boosts your adrenaline, which gets you going, but constant stress can run you down. How you manage the stresses and strains of everyday living will determine how healthy and happy you remain; reflexology can help you manage stress.

Your body is very powerful and, like nature, has its own cycles and rhythms. It can normally heal itself in its own time, but reflexology can help speed up this process. However, it is important to note that a reflexologist doesn't claim to cure your symptoms and doesn't treat a specific illness or prescribe medicines for you. This is left to medical practitioners – doctors, consultants, etc. – who are able to diagnose your symptoms. Reflexology simply works on your whole body by helping to bring it back into balance and harmony.

History

Reflexology is an ancient art, a science and a healing therapy. It has recently been rediscovered and has become very popular as a result of a need to find alternative ways to relax, to help relieve pain and to help with many different illnesses.

The Chinese are said to have used energy medicine as long ago as 3000 BC and traditionally the East has given the West many insights into how the mind, body and spirit work together to create health. The ancient Indians, Africans and Russians also practised their own methods of reflexology. Egyptian tombs depict murals and hieroglyphics in which medicine, herbs, hand and foot reflexology are being administered.

In the early twentieth century the American ear, nose and throat specialist Dr William Fitzgerald travelled to Europe and saw the practice of zone therapy, which was then being used to help with pain control. Around 1909 he did further research on the theory and divided the body into 10 vertical zones. He used instruments to put pressure on certain zones which corresponded to areas in the body where he needed to perform minor surgery and was very successful with this therapy in America.

In the 1930s another American, physiotherapist Eunice Ingham, further developed zone therapy methods. She mapped out the reflex points on the feet and their corresponding organs or areas in the body, and called it 'reflexology'. Eunice wrote two books, *Stories the Feet Can Tell* and *Stories the Feet Have Told*, which are still popular today.

One of Eunice Ingham's pupils was called Doreen Bayley. She was a pioneer in the 1960s. Doreen set up the Bayley School of Reflexology and was very influential in establishing reflexology in the UK. She too undertook her own research and drew her own reflexology maps.

Reflexology continues to evolve and today there are many different methods to this healing art. For example, it is now being practised in conjunction with other therapies, such as acupuncture (some therapists have developed reflexology using the acupuncture meridians), shiatsu, massage, etc. This is a healthy sign. However reflexology works wonders on its own!

The Self-Help Approach

Self-help means taking responsibility for yourself and learning to listen to your body and do the best you can to look after it. Life can be so hectic that it is easy to neglect yourself. Yet your most important relationship is with yourself because you need to understand, trust, listen and communicate who you are in order to relate fully to others. Reflexology can help you with this. By setting aside time to practise it on yourself you are saying that you are important and worth looking after.

Practising the self-help routines and workouts in this book can be fun and pleasurable. They can improve your life by helping to keep you happy and relaxed. Feeling safe to touch yourself also brings you more body awareness. Trust your instincts about what your body needs in order to stay healthy and happy, using a discriminative mind to decide the best course of action.

Reflexology helps to balance your whole mind, body and spirit. Your physical body needs touch, love, food and exercise, etc. Your mind needs positive mental stimulation, intellectual learning or education and a positive outlook, and your spirit needs to feel it is connected to people, to the earth and to humanity. When you practise reflexology on yourself it helps to bring out positive thinking and clarity of thought, helps you feel connected to yourself (and therefore to others) and helps your physical health; ultimately, it helps keep you balanced.

Because the reflexology works holistically, you need to work on your whole body – or on the whole of your hands or feet – before and after you practise any of the routines or workouts. So first, follow the general relaxation techniques on pages 28-29. Then you can start work on your self-help routine or workout. To begin with, you may like simply to practise the general relaxation techniques for a few days until you feel confident enough to work on yourself.

Self-help reflexology is available anywhere, anytime. Very often you may need to practise your routines away from your home – whilst travelling on a bus, train or plane, in a car (as a passenger obviously) or in the office. This is a great advantage, but in an ideal world it is always best to practise reflexology at home – in a quiet environment with soft music and with the dog, cat and children safely out of sight and the answer phone switched on. This way you can give yourself time and space to enjoy your routine, and to obtain the maximum benefits from it.

Wherever you are, remember to read the 'Dos and Don'ts Checklist' on page 34 and consult your doctor before you start work on yourself. It is also important to take responsibility for yourself and consult your doctor as soon as possible should you experience any adverse reaction to your reflexology routines or workouts.

Reflexology is a wonderful, safe and natural therapy. When you practise it with respect, it can help bring balance and harmony to your whole body, and uplift and inspire you.

HEALING

Do you ever remember being ill or bruising your knee when you were little and somebody kissing it or rubbing it better? Or have you ever had a problem and a kind person has listened to you and held your hand? They were giving you healing. Healing is natural and we all do it all the time, often without thinking. A smile from a friend really lifts you up when you are feeling low – and that keeps them smiling, too. Healing can take place in a moment, but it can influence your whole lifetime.

Healing brings about change. Although this may not always seem beneficial at the time, when you look back later you often realize the changes all happened to you for a reason. Sometimes, however, facing the truth is too painful. Many people don't heal because they are not prepared to look at the cause of their problems and let them go. Difficulties may be physical, emotional, mental or spiritual, but the principle is the same. Sometimes the letting go is also traumatic, which is why you may stay in an unsuitable job or relationship. You prefer to hold on to the pain you know because the unknown is too scary. Pain and illness themselves can become an identity which you are reluctant to let go of, particularly if you like moaning! And change doesn't always mean you get what you want; in some cases it means your physical problems may get worse. This is, however, all part of the healing process.

Life expands and contracts like your heartbeat. If you accept change and try to make the most out of every situation, then your life is able to flow freely. Resistance to change is fine for a short time, but any problem left unsolved gathers energy which can manifest into a bigger problem later on.

Energy is all around us. Have you ever seen the heat rising from a road baking in the midday sun, or seen the electrical power of a thunderstorm? This can give you an idea of just how much energy is around us all the time. According to science, objects are not solid but are moving particles of energy. The sun and moon radiate energy and in Eastern cultures people run their lives in accordance with their cycles because they believe that helps them get the most out of their lives.

Your own body is made up of energies which feed, and feed off, other energies in your environment. Energy is also referred as ch'i, yin/yang, life force, prana or vital energy; terms you may already be familiar with. Everyone and everything has its own energy field, or electromagnetic field, which is called an aura. Many people are able to see the aura with the naked eye and it can be photographed by special cameras. Your aura changes constantly in reaction to your environment and your thoughts. You body also has seven chakras or energy vortices shaped like cones which run down your spinal chord, at intervals. These metabolize and distribute energy into your body and feed the organs they govern.

The Earth itself has an aura – when it is photographed from space a blue haze can be seen around it. It also has a magnetic energy field which vibrates in waves. Healers tune into this magnetic field; when they are aligned to these energies they transmit them to help heal others. Complementary therapies, including of course reflexology, use different methods to activate these healing energies.

All energy flows and in reflexology it can be seen to flow through the 10 zones of your body. When you think badly about someone, it affects your whole body, as it can slow down your energy and stagnate it. When you think happy thoughts, on the other hand, your energies flow faster and this feeds your environment. So as you respond to your environment internally and externally, you also contribute to it. You can pollute the atmosphere by your thoughts or actions. For example, when you walk into a room where people have been arguing, you feel uncomfortable and may leave.

You will have realized that as you get tired your personal energy seems to run out and as you get older your energy levels slow down. You may also be exhausted by being under stress; if you are always on overload, your body will signal you to slow down. You can recharge your batteries by taking a walk in the park, eating, meditating, sharing a conversation with a friend, enjoying physical touch, focusing on something you love doing, exercising, breathing deeply, receiving reflexology or sleeping. During this time your body gathers energy from the vast energy source surrounding you.

Illness starts when some part of your body goes out of balance, so you may need to look at all areas of your life: are you getting enough food, touch, physical exercise? Do you partake in sharing and intimacy, socializing (emotional and physical)? Do you stimulate your mind with new information and learning (mental), and do you have a sense of belonging and being able to give to your family or community or serve the world (spiritual)? These are all areas you need to satisfy to help maintain balance.

The Aura

As already mentioned, the energy field or electromagnetic field surrounding each person is called the aura. It comprises seven levels of energy. Each level is called an energy body. The first level is the physical body, the second the emotional body, etc. Each vibrates at a different rate and the physical body vibrates the slowest. On Earth our vibration is quite slow; trees and flowers have faster vibrations than humans. Each energy body affects the rest and when a number of them go out of sync at once your physical health can be affected. Many illnesses begin in the upper levels of the aura and gradually work down to the physical body. Therefore it is important that you keep your aura clear and flowing. Reflexology helps you to do this by stimulating the energies in your aura and moving 'negative' or stagnant energies out of your body.

You can feel your own aura and sense other people's. For example, when people get too close to you without your permission you may feel that your personal space has been invaded.

Let's look at each energy body in turn.

1ST LEVEL – PHYSICAL BODY

This level of your aura is found up to 2.5cm (1") from your physical body and is generally a misty grey-blue colour. If you have a strong physical body, feel physically safe and comfortable, have vitality and like physical touch and sex, then this level will be healthy. If you feel insecure, avoid physical touch or physical intimacy, and are dreamy and ungrounded, then your physical body may be out of balance.

2ND LEVEL – EMOTIONAL BODY

Your emotional body lies around 7.5 cm (3") from your physical body and can sometimes be seen as watery pastel colours. When this body is healthy and balanced you feel calm and good about yourself, feel self-love and love for others, and are able to express your emotions positively. When it is out of balance you may feel negative emotions which you may not be able to express in a positive way or you may feel totally cut off from your emotions.

3RD LEVEL – MENTAL BODY

It is possible for some people to see this level of the aura, usually a yellow colour, around 23cm (9") from your physical body. When your mental body is healthy, you are able to think clearly, have a strong mind and need mental stimulation in your life. When this body is out of balance you may be unfocused and confused, have mental problems or be a pessimistic thinker.

4TH LEVEL – ASTRAL BODY

This is around 35cm (14") from your physical body and is made of up a variety of colours. When your astral body is healthy you are able to have healthy and intimate relationships with people, and you may enjoy working for your community. If this body is out of balance you may avoid intimate relationships.

5TH LEVEL – IMPRESSION BODY

This body usually looks dark blue and lies around 61cm (2') from your physical body and is dark in colour. When the impression body is balanced, you are aligned to your life purpose. If you are disconnected from your life purpose, you may reject boundaries and structure or be very disorganized. Then this level is out of balance.

6TH LEVEL – WISDOM BODY

This body can be seen as an array of iridescent colours around 1m (3.5') from your physical body. When it is balanced, it brings joy, peace, healing, a feeling of connection, love and harmony. When it is out of balance, you may reject any form of spiritual connection.

7TH LEVEL – SPIRITUAL BODY

This lies about 1.21cm (4') from your physical body and makes a golden egg shape around it. When it is healthy you will have great clarity about your spirituality. You may be telepathic, introspective and search for the truth within, and you may view the world as a whole. When this level is blocked or out of balance you may be impatient, a perfectionist and a dreamer who feels isolated and cut off from the world.

The Chakras

As well as the seven energy bodies surrounding you there are also seven chakras, or spinning vortices of energy, which lie along your spinal cord at points where there are a gathering of nerves,

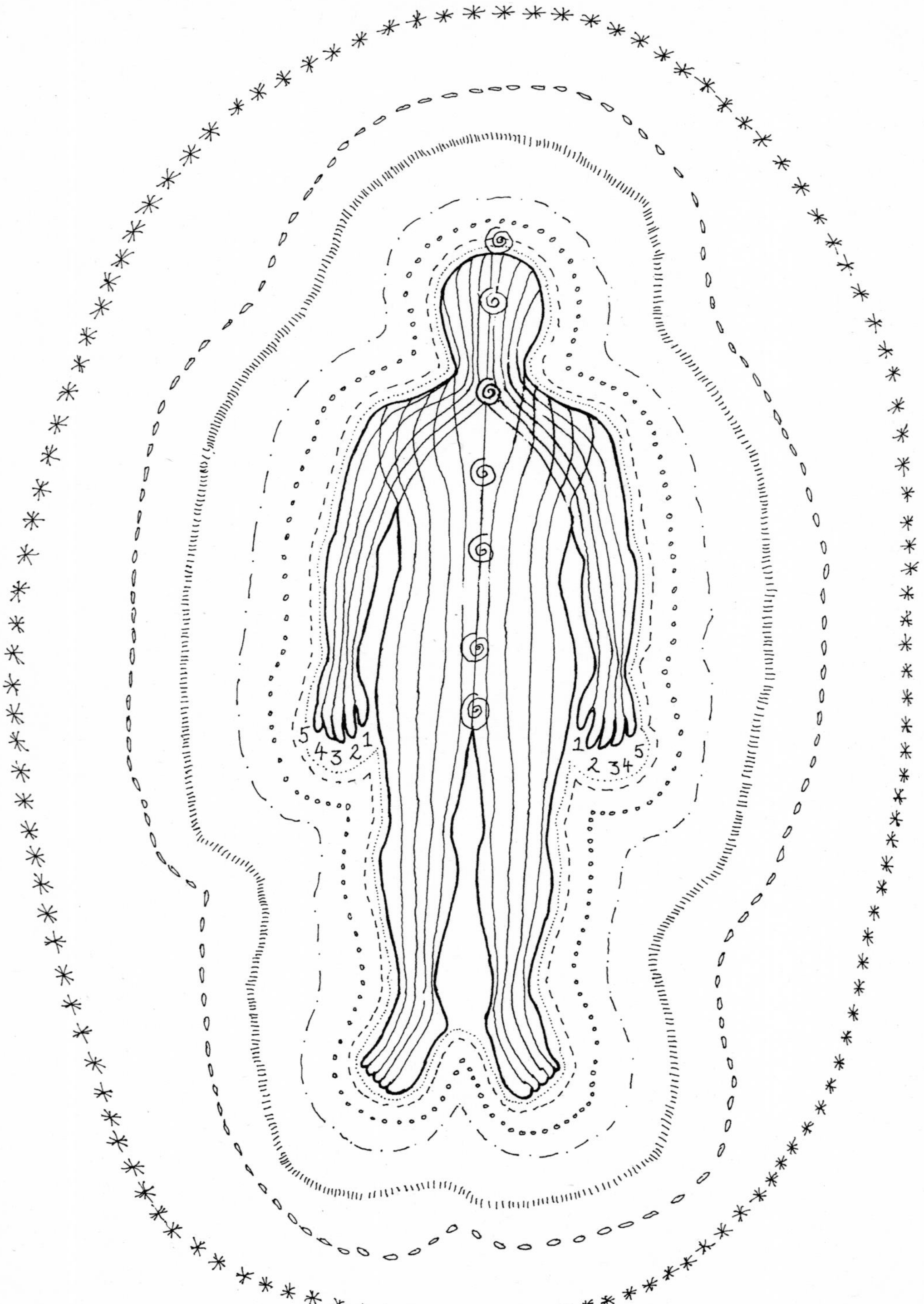
5 4 3 2 1
1 2 3 4 5

taking in energy and feeding it to the organs governing each area.

BASE CHAKRA – RED

Found between your legs, this chakra supplies energy to your adrenal glands, kidneys, intestines, pelvis, hips, legs and feet, and is associated with touch and your sense of survival.

SACRAL CHAKRA – ORANGE

Situated around 2" below your navel, this chakra supplies energy to your reproductive organs and lower back, and

---

Left: The human aura, chakras and the 10 zones of the body

KEY

THE AURA

✳ ✳ ✳ PHYSICAL BODY

◡ ◡ ◡ ◡ EMOTIONAL BODY

/川∪//川∪//川∪// MENTAL BODY

‒ ‒ · ‒ · ‒ ASTRAL BODY

o o o o o o o IMPRESSION BODy

· ‒ ‒ · ‒ WISDOM BODY

· · · · · · · · · · · SPIRITUAL BODY

(�) CHAKRAS (from head to toe)

7 CROWN CHAKRA, purple

6 EYE CHAKRA, indigo

5 THROAT CHAKRA, blue

4 HEART CHAKRA, green or pink

3 SOLAR PLEXUS CHAKRA, yellow

2 SACRAL CHAKRA, orange

1 BASE CHAKRA, red

---

is associated with sexuality, sensuality and the immune system.

SOLAR PLEXUS CHAKRA – YELLOW

You can find this chakra in your middle, just below your diaphragm. It supplies energy to your gall bladder, liver, intestines, pancreas, spleen, stomach, diaphragm, middle back and entire nervous system. It helps you to relate to others.

HEART CHAKRA – GREEN OR PINK

This lies in your heart area and metabolizes energy to keep your heart, circulatory system, upper back and thymus healthy. Love, compassion, affection and caring are associated with this chakra.

THROAT CHAKRA – BLUE

Found in your throat area, this chakra energizes your thyroid, lungs, neck, ears, nose, mouth and teeth. Hearing, taste and self-expression through communication of your truth are associated with this chakra.

EYE CHAKRA – INDIGO

Situated between your eyes, this supplies vital energy to your pituitary gland, eyes, face, brain and nervous system. It is involved with your understanding of ideas and your ability to trust your instincts.

CROWN CHAKRA – PURPLE

Your crown chakra is found of the top of your head and supplies energy to your pineal gland and upper brain. It is involved with your ability to face reality and your sense of 'knowing'.

THE SYSTEMS OF THE BODY

In order for you to understand how your body works the following section describes the nine main systems and the organs of your body. It is useful to have a brief reminder of what we are made up of! The numbers in brackets refer to points featured on Jim Horan's reflexology charts (see pages 115 to 119).

The Circulatory System

Your circulatory system is made up of your heart **16**, blood vessels and blood. Your arteries and blood capillaries carry oxygenated blood and nutrients to every cell in your body, whilst your veins carry blood containing carbon dioxide (de-oxygenated blood) back through your heart to your lungs for oxygenation. This helps detoxify your body.

Everyone also belongs to one of four different blood groups: A, B, AB and O. It is useful to know which, should you ever need to receive or give blood. There is also a substance in your blood called the Rhesus factor (Rh); most people are Rh positive and fewer people Rh negative.

The circulatory system provides your cells with oxygen, vitamins and minerals, hormones and antibodies to wherever they are needed, in order to help maintain your body in optimum health.

Common complaints of this system are heart attack, blood pressure imbalances, varicose veins and the rare hereditary disease haemophilia, where the blood refuses to clot.

The Digestive System

Your digestive system comprises your teeth **2**, **43**, mouth **2**, **43**, tongue **43**, salivary glands, oesophagus, stomach **22**, duodenum **24**, pancreas **25**, small intestine **42**, large intestine **30**, **32**, **33**, **34**, **37**, liver **19** and gall bladder **23**. Its function is to take in food and change it into absorbable substances for your body to use and then to eliminate any waste products. From beginning to end, your digestive tract is over 10m long!

Some of the problems associated with your digestive system are constipation, diarrhoea, irritable bowel syndrome, ulcers, allergies and heartburn.

The Endocrine System

Your pituitary **5**, pineal **4**, thyroid **12**, parathyroid **12**, thymus **50**, adrenal **26**, pancreas **25**, ovaries **44** and testes **44** are all ductless glands that secrete hormones directly into your bloodstream. The hormones are then circulated throughout your body to help keep your chemical and emotional balance. Hormones are also used for healthy growth and for sexual development.

Ovarian cysts, fibroids, emotional instability, infertility, thyroid and blood sugar imbalances are diseases of your endocrine system. Premenstrual tension, ranging from carelessness and irritability to headaches and nausea, is caused when your hormone levels become imbalanced around menstruation.

The Lymphatic System

This system functions like a secondary circulatory system. It is made up of lymph vessels and ducts, lymph nodes, lymph fluid, the spleen **28**, tonsils **8**, adenoids, thymus gland **50** and appendix **39**. Its function is to protect your body from infection.

Breast problems like lumps, mastitis and cancer are diseases of your lymphatic system, along with any type of infection and cancers which can affect the lymphatic system. Also 'auto-immune' diseases, whereby your body's immune system starts to react to and destroy its own tissues, are associated with this system.

The Muscular System

Your muscular system contains around 640 different muscles, which are supplied with arteries (which carry oxygenated blood to them) and veins (which take away waste products like carbon dioxide).

Your muscles make up around half of your body weight and are divided into two different categories: voluntary and involuntary. Voluntary muscles are used with awareness and conscious thought when running, walking, gardening, etc. They are never completely relaxed; this is called 'muscle tone'. Involuntary muscles are used without any conscious awareness; they help run your heart **16**, intestinal wall **30**, **31**, **32**, **33**, **34**, **37** and diaphragm **18**, etc.

Every hair on your body has a muscle attached to it which helps regulate your body temperature. When you are cold or scared each hair is pulled up by its muscles, causing 'goose flesh'.

Cramp is a common complaint of the muscular system; it happens when two opposing muscles contract at once. Backache, muscle strains, muscular stiffness and muscles spasms are other problems that may be experienced.

The Nervous System

This system is divided into the central nervous system and autonomous nervous system, both containing nerves which are used to communicate messages from your brain to all parts of your body, and from your body to your brain. Your brain **1**, spinal cord **52**-**56** and solar plexus **17** are all part of your nervous system.

Neuralgia is a common complaint of this system. It causes local pain due to inflammation or exposure of nerves (for instance a tooth which has lost its filling). Sciatica, a complaint which often brings chronic lower back pain, is caused by inflammation of the sciatic nerve, which runs from the lower back to your legs.

The Reproductive System

In women the reproductive system comprises the vagina, uterus **45**, Fallopian tubes **46**, ovaries **44** and mammary glands; in men, the penis, seminal vesicles **46**, vas deferens **46**, prostate **45** and testes **44**. This system is used to produce and, in women, carry a new baby.

One complaint of the reproductive system is an ectopic pregnancy, where a foetus situates itself outside your womb, for example in a Fallopian tube, instead of in your uterus.

The Respiratory System

This consists of the upper respiratory system – your nose **51**, vocal cords, throat **8**, larynx and sinuses **2** – and the lower respiratory system – the windpipe, bronchi and lungs **13**, alveoli, or air sacs, and diaphragm **18**. It functions by breathing in oxygenated air (to inspire) and breathing out carbon dioxide and a little water (to expire). This helps detoxify your body.

Asthma and bronchitis are common ailments of your respiratory system. Bronchitis is a condition where your lung tissues are inflamed due to infection or sometimes the inhalation of fumes or chemicals.

The Skeletal System

The adult skeletal system has approximately 206 bones in it. They provide a frame for your body and a framework for all your other systems. Some bones (your skull, pelvic bones, spinal column and rib cage) are also used specifically to protect your organs. Your bones are also used to achieve movement. They are made up of around 45 per cent minerals, 30 per cent organic materials and 25 per cent water. The long bones in your body contain bone marrow, which makes red blood cells to carry oxygen around the system, and white blood cells, which make up the immune system.

Curvature of the spine is one of the diseases found in your skeletal system. Bones can also break or fracture.

The Urinary System

Your kidneys **27**, ureters **32** (two tubes which carry urine from your kidneys to your bladder), bladder **36** and urethra are all part of your urinary system. Their job is to filter out waste products from your body.

Kidney stones and cystitis are common diseases of this system, cystitis being when your bladder becomes inflamed as a result of infection. This can cause a burning sensation when you urinate, and sometimes acute pain and a high temperature. Kidney infections are usually caused by an infection from your bladder travelling up your ureters to your kidneys. Such infections can be very serious and can reoccur if not cleared up properly or if you have weak kidneys.

LOOKING AFTER YOUR FEET

Your feet have a very important job to perform – they carry you through life and help you balance and stay upright. You can really ruin your feet with ill-fitting shoes that compress and suppress your circulation and bones into restricting spaces. Then you are more likely to get problems like corns and calluses, blisters and even deformity. However it can be more complicated than this, because your feet mirror every part of your body and having problems with your feet can affect your health. Similarly if you have a problem with any part of your body, you may suddenly notice more hard skin growing in that reflex area on your hands or feet afterwards.

Common Conditions of the Feet

CORNS

Corns are hard or thickened skin which are cone shaped and tend to pop up from something rubbing them, like new or ill-fitting shoes. You find them around the joints of your toes or on the heel or ball of your feet, where there is a lot of friction. Sometimes they can become extremely painful, so you may like to visit a chiropodist to get them removed.

ATHLETE'S FOOT

This is a fungal infection which usually materializes on the skin between your toes, which becomes patchy, flaky and itchy. It is contagious and you can catch it from public places like swimming pools, saunas or gymnasiums, or anywhere you don't wear shoes.

BUNIONS

Bunions are caused by swelling that builds up around a joint in order to protect it from friction. The swelling often takes place around your metatarsal joint where it meets your big toe and is very painful as it rubs against your shoes. Going barefoot can help take the pressure off, or you can have it removed if it prevents you from walking properly.

CALLUS

This is hard skin which build ups anywhere on the soles of your feet (but very often around your heels) caused by the constant pressure of walking or standing on them. Regular reflexology can help prevent this. You can also buy foot creams and rough nail files from your chemist to help remove it or if it is very thick or painful you can have it removed by a chiropodist.

FLAT FEET

Flat feet occur as a result of weakness in your joints from being overweight or from general weakness in your body (particularly in childhood), or may be hereditary. The condition can affect your whole health because it puts strain on your spine. Arch supports are often recommended by chiropodists to help.

ARCHED FEET

Arched feet are often hereditary. The unusually high arch prevents your ball and toes from connecting or grounding with the earth. If you choose, you can have an operation to correct this problem.

PART 1

How To Use Self-Help Reflexology

WARMING UP

Giving yourself reflexology can be a very pleasurable experience, uplifting, relaxing and stimulating your whole body. Warming up, or setting the environment for your reflexology routine, is very important because it helps you to feel comfortable and get the maximum benefits from your efforts. Setting the environment means preparing your inner self, too, bringing your awareness to where you are and what you're doing.

Preparation
Remember to cut or file your fingernails so that they don't scratch or dig in whilst you're working and find a blanket to wrap around you in case you get cold. Make sure you wash your hands and/or feet or use antiseptic wipes on them before you start your routine, then apply (preferably aluminium-free) talcum powder, an aqueous cream or a base oil like almond oil. You may also like to get a glass of water ready to drink when you've finished.

Creating the Ideal Setting
Ideally, you are going to practise your routine at home, either at the beginning or end of the day if you go out to work, or sometime during the day if you are at home. However, it's not always possible to practise in an ideal setting because you may be at work, travelling or in an outside environment. The main thing, wherever you are, is to try to relax – if you know you've left your car on a parking meter that's just about to run out, for instance, you are not going to be able to give yourself your full attention! Try to let all other distractions go.

Sound: Give yourself space; make sure all your pets and children are happily and safely engaged elsewhere if possible. If your children suddenly decide to descend upon you when you are in the middle of your routine or your dog starts to bark because it is hungry, you are not going to be able to relax properly. Make sure you turn the telephone off or put your answer phone on so there aren't any outside distractions. You may like to play some soft music or you may prefer perfect peace.

Scent: You may like to burn some lavender oil in an aromatherapy burner in your room, have sweet-smelling flowers near you or open the window (if it's warm) and smell fresh air as you practise reflexology. Having sensual smells around you can really make you feel good.

Sight: Colours are very important and can greatly affect your mood. Generally cool colours such as greens and blues calm you down and warm colours such as reds and pinks stimulate you. Having pleasurable colours around you whilst you are practising your routine can help you to relax. You may also like to sit by a window or even in your garden if it is quiet, so that you feel connected to nature and enjoy the natural colours around you.

Taste: You can taste water after your session or a herbal tea if you prefer to refresh you and stimulate your taste buds as well as help expel toxins.

Touch: Touch can be very nurturing, and feeling safe to touch yourself, feeling comfortable with your body, helps you to relax. You may hardly ever touch your feet and therefore it can be exciting and interesting to explore this unknown area of your body.

Breathing

Breathing is very important; it helps detoxify your body. You inhale oxygen into your lungs and exhale stale air from them. Most people breathe shallowly, particularly when stressed. If you don't breathe properly, you are unable to get the most out of your life or function at 100 per cent because you are not energizing your body. Your breathing is affected by pollution, stuffy rooms and atmospheres, dust, pollen, etc. Each time you breathe in you are breathing more life and vital energies into your body.

Breathing can help relax you and simple breathing exercises can help calm and re-energize you when you are feeling scattered, off balance or tired. Breathing also helps you stay in the moment and allows you to simply 'be' with your body, not in the past or the future, but just where you are right now!

You may like to try the following simple breathing exercise for a few minutes before practising your reflexology routines or workouts.

Close your eyes and lie or sit down in a comfortable position with your spine straight. Be aware of the breath going in and out of your mouth. Next bring your awareness to you abdomen and concentrate on the breath going in and out of that area. You can even place one hand on your abdomen and feel it rising and falling as you breathe in and out. Don't force anything. Simply give all your attention to your in-breath and out-breath.

Sometimes you may notice that you breathe in longer than you breathe out, or vice versa. Enjoy being with yourself and feeling relaxed.

Preparing for Others

Your friends and family may ask you to practise on them as a result of seeing how beneficial reflexology has been for you, but wait until you have practised your routines many times and feel confident before you do this. Remember they must visit their doctor to check whether it is safe for them to receive reflexology before you work on them. Go through the 'Dos and Don'ts Checklist' with them as well.

If you are practising on them in their home environment, you can help them to get the most out of it by making it as relaxed as possible too. Always ask the person you are practising on what they would like to do (and not what you think would be best for them to do) whilst preparing their environment to help them relax.

Making the Most of Reflexology outside your Home

If you get a splitting headache at the office it is not going to be ideal to practise there but it can help. Try to find a quiet corner away from bright lights, take some gentle breaths, work the general relaxation techniques before and after you practise self-help reflexology.

Wherever you are – on a bus, plane, train, at work or in the countryside – do the best you can and be adaptable to your environment whilst practising your routines and workouts.

REFLEXOLOGY TECHNIQUES

Before and after you practise any of your self-help routines it is important that you practise the general relaxation techniques, numbered one to three overleaf, for a few minutes to work on your whole body. Then you can apply the further techniques, numbered four to nine, to experiment and add variety to your routines and workouts.

Remember to work your reflex points carefully and don't press too hard or work too long because you may overstimulate the areas of your body you are working on.

Also, stay within the time allocated for each routine. When you first start you may find that you are not fast enough to fit your routines into the time allocated. This is OK; it may take a while for you to get familiar with your body and its reflexes. A good way to work up your confidence is to get really comfortable with the basic movements illustrated below before you attempt any of the self-help routines or workouts.

Find out what pressure suits you when you are working on your hands or feet (or somebody else's); you may like it firm but others may like a light, gentle pressure, and vice versa. You may also find that you vary the pressure you use each time you practise; this is quite common. Finding the best pressure for you each time means that you will feel more comfortable during your routine, which in turn will help you to relax and really enjoy your reflexology.

You will know that you have found areas that are out of balance because they may feel sensitive, sore, sharp or spongy, or you may feel crystal deposits or gritty bits. These are the blockages in your energy flow.

Practising reflexology is easy once you know your way around your body on your hands and feet, but whilst you are learning you may fumble and overconcentrate. This makes it harder work, but be patient, be playful, trust yourself and have fun!

GENERAL RELAXATION TECHNIQUES

1 The Caterpillar Walk

The basic reflexology technique is achieved by using
your thumb or first finger in a caterpillar movement.
To do this, *press* your finger or thumb in to the skin,
slide the thumb forward a little, and *press* again.
Work your way across each area like this, in a
caterpillar walk.

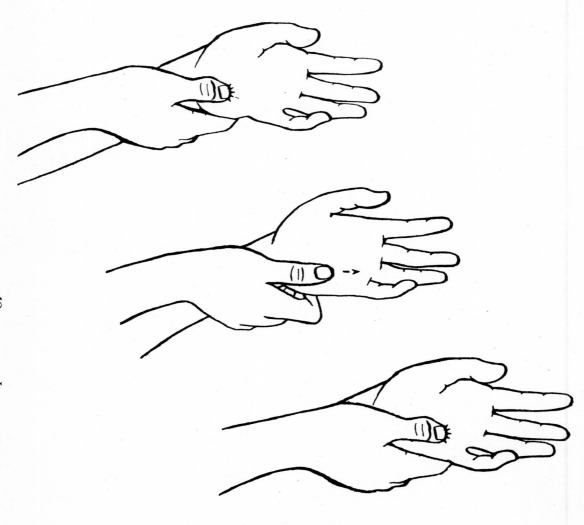

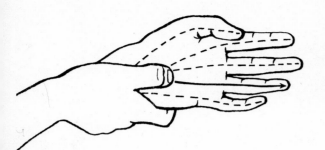

2 The caterpillar walking the five zones

Next, use your caterpillar movement (*press*, *slide*, *press*) to walk up the five zones of the soles of each foot or palms of each hand (including your toes and fingers). Then walk *across* each hand or foot. Be gentle when working over your tendons.

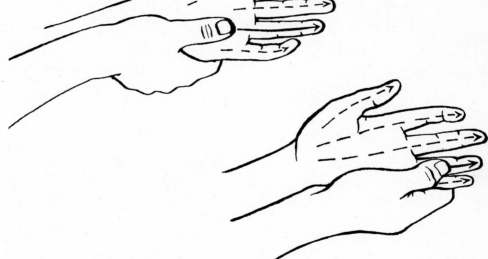

3 Solar plexus movement

Next locate your solar plexus reflex point on each hand. These correspond to the knotted feeling you get around your middle when you are tense or stressed. Press your thumb into these areas and add pressure, then release.

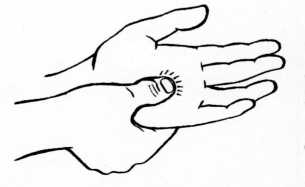

General Relaxation

You can add any of the following techniques to your general relaxation techniques. Remember to always work with care – if any movement feels uncomfortable, alter the pressure. See which movements you like best …

4 The Hook

Keeping your hand at right angles to the foot or hand that you are working on, simply use your thumb to hook into your reflex points. This technique is particularly used on the pituitary gland.

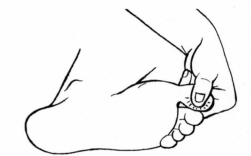

5 Kneading

You can use the knuckles of your hand to knead the soles of your feet or the palms of your hands. Use a light to medium pressure.

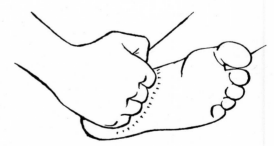

6 Chopping

Using the side of your fingers, lightly slap the palms of your hands.

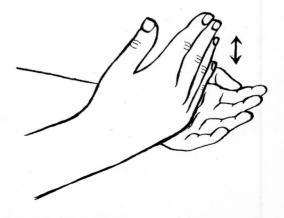

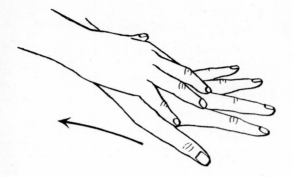

7 Stroking

Using a very light touch, allow your fingers to stroke your feet or hands from your toes towards your heels (or your fingertips towards your wrist). Make sure you stroke in only one direction.

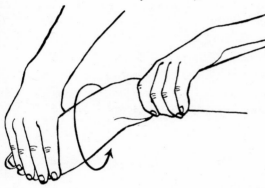

8 Rotating

Support your ankle or wrist with one hand and gently rotate your foot or hand clockwise and anti-clockwise with your other hand, using smooth movements.

9 Toe Twirling

Hold each of your toes individually whilst supporting your foot with your other hand and gently twirl each around clockwise.

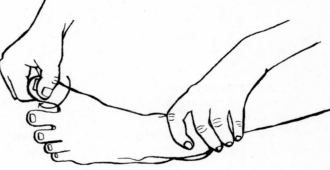

AFTERWARDS

It's best not to rush around immediately after your routine or workout. Spend a few minutes breathing gently and quietly before moving. Drink a glass of water.

HOW WILL IT MAKE ME FEEL?

Your body is completely different from everyone else's and so your response to reflexology will also differ from that of the next person. Even your own reaction to it will be different from one day to the next because your body is constantly changing. One day you may feel mentally alert and energetic with a sense of well-being, the next you may feel tired and emotional.

If you have a cold or other infection, you may feel tired after practising reflexology or your cold may seem as though it is getting worse for a short time because of the toxins rising to the surface to be released from your body. If you are working on the routine for sleeplessness, you may feel more alert afterwards or you may feel sleepy because your body needs more rest. Remember, your body knows what it needs to bring it back into balance. It's best to be free of expectations about how your body may react to reflexology.

However in most cases you will feel more relaxed after reflexology and if you are under stress it can help you to face the world again. Remember the reflexology routines and workouts in this book are aimed at helping you to manage your body and to take responsibility for your life, rather than cure you of your ills. Below is a list of some of the general reactions you may experience after practising self-help reflexology:

Physical
You may be:
Energetic (from stimulating your body)
Tired (from the release of toxins)
Sweaty (from increased circulation)
Shaky (from release or increase of nervous energy)
Dizzy (from oxygenation of your body)
Nauseous (from the release of toxins)
You may have:
Darker urine (from release of toxins)
Altered heartbeat (as your breathing balances out)
A skin rash (from release of toxins through your skin)
An increase in vaginal discharge (from stimulation of your hormones)
Bowel movements (from balancing of your digestive system)
Headaches (from the release of toxins)

Emotional
You may feel:
Weepy (from a release of emotions)
Good (from a feeling of well-being)
Happy, calm and balanced emotionally
Over-emotional (from releasing stress)

Mental
You may have:
Mental clarity
Confusion
Mental alertness
Indifference

Spiritual
You may feel:
Connected to life and others
An inner self-awareness
Spiritual peace (from inner connection with self)
No connection to spirituality

If you do have one or more reactions, feel glad that you are experiencing the release of negative energies which may have been causing illness or lying in wait to cause problems later on. Reactions usually pass away quite quickly, but if they continue, or if you are worried by any reaction, then talk about it to your doctor. However, normally any reaction following reflexology is nothing to be alarmed about. A reaction may not appear for some hours after your reflexology routine or may appear immediately.

If you have no reaction at all, that's fantastic. Don't worry, it does not mean that reflexology hasn't worked! We all have different reactions to experience. Have fun getting to know yourself!

DOS AND DON'TS CHECKLIST

Reflexology is a very safe, natural therapy which has been practised for thousands of years, and today is used in many health centres, hospitals and clinics all over the world. When you practise reflexology with care and consideration you will feel wonderful and reap its benefits. However, please remember to follow the basic guidelines as laid out in this checklist. If you are practising a routine on a friend or family member, make sure you go through this information with them carefully.

It is recommended that you consult your doctor before receiving or practising reflexology. Your doctor particularly needs to know if you have any suspected illness, recurrent or undiagnosed pain, are pregnant, on medication, or have recently had an operation, and will consult your medical history before assessing whether it is safe for you to receive reflexology. It may be better for you to see a professional reflexologist for treatment rather than practising on yourself.

DOS:

- DO remember to practise the general relaxation techniques for a few minutes before and after practising any of the self-help routines in this book.

- DO make sure that you cover up any verrucaes on your feet with a plaster to prevent spreading infection.

- DO use a very gentle pressure on yourself if you have osteoporosis, fragile bones, are menstruating, or have any inflammation or swelling on your feet or hands.

- DO try to keep your back straight when you practise self-help reflexology, to avoid backache from poor posture.

- DO use a very gentle pressure when you are working on the elderly or young children.

- DO remember to drink a glass of water after your routine.

- DO remember to consult your doctor if you are worried about any reaction you may have as a result of receiving reflexology.

DON'TS:

- DON'T receive reflexology if you are less than four months pregnant or if you are prone to miscarriage.

- DON'T work on the reflexes for your reproductive organs (ovaries, uterus, Fallopian tubes) or pituitary gland during pregnancy.

- DON'T receive reflexology if you have phlebitis or thrombosis.

- DON'T work directly over any injured bones, cuts, bruises, scar tissue or damaged areas.

- DON'T work over varicose veins.

- DON'T work over athlete's foot, otherwise you may spread the infection.

- DON'T practise more than one self-help routine or workout in one day; only practise for the length of time allocated.

PART 2

Self-Help for Energy and Vitality

THE SELF-HELP WORKOUTS

Regular reflexology can help serve as preventative healthcare, helping to oppose the ageing process by releasing tension from your body and by detoxifying it to keep you healthy. It can bring you energy and vitality. Let reflexology inspire you to appreciate your amazing body (even if you don't think it's perfect) and the job it does in carrying you through life and allowing you to experience it. Learn to make friends with yourself as you work on your routines and enjoy touching yourself. Touch helps you to feel secure, to feel safe and comfortable in your skin. It is very healing – and can help make you beautiful too!

The energy and vitality workouts are designed for you to get the most out of your life by helping you to feel beautiful and happy. Feeling good on the inside can make you feel and look beautiful on the outside.

So it is important to let go of stress, because stress can cause you to look ugly: lines around your face, a lack of vitality, dull complexion and hair, etc. Learn to face your fears and accept change. The more you learn to adapt to and accept your circumstances in life the more beautiful you'll stay. Learn to laugh at life, even in the bad times – it will get you through and help prevent problems from draining your energy and vitality.

Remember to consult your doctor before practising any of your self-help workouts and read the 'Dos and Don'ts Checklist' on page 34. Read 'Warming Up' (page 25), then practise your general relaxation techniques (page 28) before and after practising any of your workouts.

The first workout is for *positive thinking* for increased confidence. Confidence means you feel good in your body and can face any situation, knowing that you are able to do the best you can, that you'll get through it. Confidence means you feel comfortable with who you are and believe in yourself. It offers you a positive outlook on life. When you are confident, you attract people because you feel more beautiful.

Even when you are confident, however, there may be times in your life when you need to practise the *strength workout* to help you get through life's ups and downs. This helps give you stamina and determination to carry on in times of distress, or when you are generally feeling tired. You may like to practise this routine to help you cope with your duties.

The *relaxation workout* has been designed to help you generally unwind at the weekend, on holiday or anytime to make you feel wonderful, sensual, relaxed and good all over.

You can work on the *vitality workout* to help inspire you and boost your energies to find that sparkle in your eye that attracts and makes you feel alive inside.

The *sex workout* can help you unwind from your day, help relax you and help you feel connected to yourself and your partner, so preparing your body for intimacy and sharing. Reflexology connects you with the same energies that you give and receive during sex.

The *metabolism workout* can help to balance your metabolism, and generally help you to feel happy in yourself so that your body finds its own healthy weight and shape.

The *detoxification workout* has been designed to help keep your body shining with health and clear of toxins. When you are healthy your body energies flow easily – and so does your whole life.

The aim of all the energy and vitality workouts is to uplift and inspire you, and to help you to love and accept your body. When you feel loved you are more lovable and are better able to share with others.

Reflexology works by helping to bring your whole body into harmony and balance. Balance is the key to a happy and healthy life, so you also need to find balance between your masculine and feminine energies. The left side of your brain and right side of your body are associated with logic, action, ambition, drive, standing up for yourself, giving and going out into the world; we call these your 'masculine' energies. When you have illnesses down this side of your body it can be a little reminder of problems with your masculinity, relationships with your father or men in general.

The right side of your brain and left side of your body are connected with creativity, receptiveness, nurturing and intuition, and these are associated with your 'feminine' energies. If you always get illness in this side of your body, then examine your relationship towards your femininity, your ability to care and nurture yourself and others, and your relationship to your mother or women in general.

Keeping the balance between your own masculine and feminine energies helps keep you happy. Today men and women's roles have become much more flexible: women often go out to work whilst men stay in and cook and look after the children. The woman is using her masculine energies to take action and provide the security, and the man being nurturing and creative. However, everyone can be both. Sometimes when we have one quality 'missing' (or dormant), we look for it in a partner or friends so that we make a whole. It is very important to be whole in yourself – and, as already mentioned, the most important relationship you have is with yourself. Practising your self-help workouts can help you to communicate with yourself to help you explore both your masculine and your feminine energies.

It is difficult to be totally self-sufficient in every area of your life, as we all have needs, which we look to other people to help us fulfil.

Mind, Body and Spirit
Reflexology can help the mind, body and spirit by giving energy and vitality.

Mind
Your workouts help your mind by encouraging positive thinking to help you accept your problems and to give you the clarity of mind to see what decisions need to be made in your life. They stimulate you to seek out knowledge, information and education or learning.

A positive attitude helps improve your quality of life. When you are negative and destructive, things tend to go wrong, your energy decreases and you become stagnant.

Body

Practising reflexology helps to keep your energies flowing and your body free from illness by eliminating toxins and keeping your whole physical body balanced. It helps your body to heal itself, giving you shining hair, clear skin, bright eyes and an energetic body brimming with vitality.

Spirit

When you practise your workouts for energy and vitality you are opening up to yourself – connecting with your inner self. When you feel connected inside it helps you to feel connected to others, even to the whole of humanity. It encourages you to think of how you can help others, serve them in some way.

 Each hand symbol represents 5 minutes duration.

1 This symbol refers to the numbered reflexology points which correspond to parts of the body as marked on Jim Horan's Easy Reference Charts on pages 114-119. Please refer to these charts for an accurate location of the reflex points. Please note that certain reflex points, for example **16** the heart and heart related areas, are located in more than one area of the hand or foot.

The Positive Thinking Workout

 TIME: 15 minutes, up to 3 times per week, on your hands. Practise the general relaxation techniques on pp 28-29 for a few minutes before and after this workout.

You will be working the following reflex areas on both hands:

1 **The brain and head** `1`
Working these points helps give you clarity of thought and alleviate worry.

2 **The throat** `8`
This reflex enables you to express yourself when lacking confidence.

3 **The pituitary gland** `5`
You can work this point firmly, to help balance your hormones to make you feel good and get you in touch with your emotions.

4 **The chest, lungs** `13` **and diaphragm** `18`
To help you to breathe deeply – when you are feeling fearful your breathing becomes very shallow and you may feel dizzy.

5 **The adrenal glands** `26`
To help calm you when you are anxious and boost your energy.

6 **The solar plexus** `17`
To help relax your nerves.

For a complete guide to the numbered points refer to the easy reference charts on pp 115-119

COMPLAINT

If you lack confidence, you may feel a sense of hopelessness, anger or lethargy, or be unhappy, insecure or fearful. You may be lazy, your creativity may be blocked and you may be unable to think positively or communicate freely.

CAUSE

This may be caused by fear of change, a reluctance to move forward with your life because you fear the unknown. You may be afraid of rejection or of not being good enough. You may not value yourself or other people may have told you you were useless, so you don't try. But this only compounds your feelings of inadequacy and results in you feeling lethargic. A lack in confidence can also be an excuse for not taking responsibility for your life.

HOW REFLEXOLOGY HELPS

Reflexology helps you connect with your inner self. Things may not always go your way, of course, but with confidence you can accept life and make the most out of it. When you radiate confidence you draw positive people and situations to you, so life improves anyway!

Physically, reflexology helps you by opening up your diaphragm to relax your breathing. This helps you 'take a deep breath and jump in at the deep end' when necessary. Reflexology works on your throat to help you express yourself, on your hormones to make you feel good, on your brain to help give you clarity about life and boosts your whole energies to increase creativity.

Self-Help for Energy and Vitality

1 The brain and head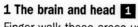

Finger walk these areas using the caterpillar movement.

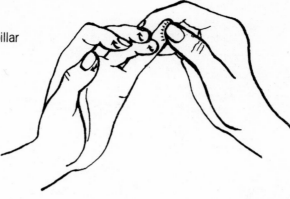

2 The throat 8

Caterpillar walk over this area using your thumb.

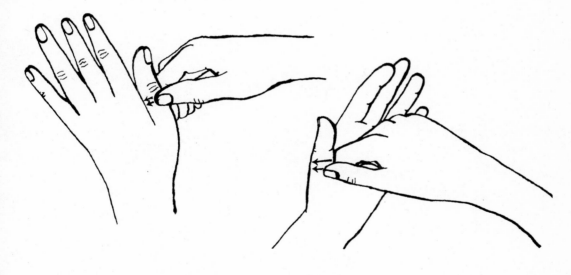

3 The pituitary gland 5

Use the hook movement, keeping your hand at right angles to these reflex points.

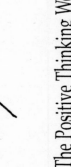

4 The chest, lungs 13 and diaphragm 18
Caterpillar walk over these areas across your hand.

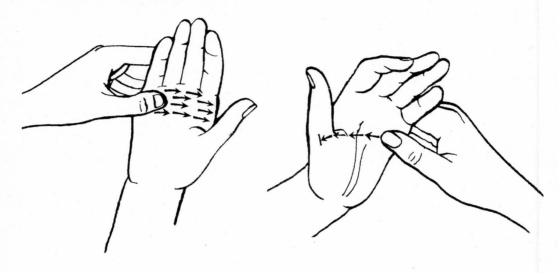

5 The adrenal glands 26
Caterpillar walk over this point.

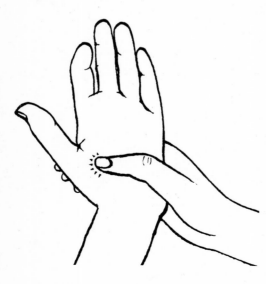

6 The solar plexus 17
Work with your thumb into this area, adding pressure then releasing. Repeat a few times.

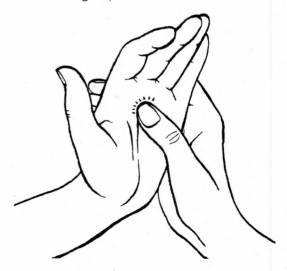

The Strength Workout

 **TIME:** 20 minutes, up to twice a week, on your hands. Practise the general relaxation techniques on pp 28-29 for a few minutes before and after this workout.

You will be working the following reflex areas on both hands:

1 **The brain and head** `1`
To help clear your mind of any confusion.

2 **The pituitary gland** `5`
To help calm your emotions and make you feel good.

3 **The thyroid gland** `12`
To help balance your metabolism.

4 **The lungs** `13` **and diaphragm** `18`
To help regulate your breathing and detoxify your body.

5 **The adrenal glands** `26`
To help balance your energy levels.

6 **The solar plexus** `17`
To help calm your nerves and relax you.

7 **The kidneys** `27`
To help eliminate toxins from your body.

8 **The spine** `52`, `53`, `54`, `56`
To help boost your circulation and relax your entire body.

9 **The sacro-ileac joint** `55`
To help relax your lower back.

For a complete guide to the numbered points refer to the easy reference charts on pp 115-119

COMPLAINT:
When you experience a lack of strength you may feel exhausted, despondent, confused, frustrated or hopeless, or be emotional and touchy. You may not feel like getting out of bed in the morning or be unable to find the will to get through another day.

CAUSE:
You may be overwhelmed by the challenges that life is throwing at you, trying to do your best but being ground down by your burdens and responsibilities. You may experience a lack of physical stamina or strength as a result of refusing to look at a problem, burying your head and denying its existence. At times in life when you see no apparent direction to go in you can also experience a loss of strength and vitality. You can also lose your strength as a result of having to be a pillar of strength for others.

HOW REFLEXOLOGY HELPS:
Reflexology can bring you inner strength by reconnecting you with your body and allowing you space and time on your own, to heal yourself. Practising your workout can help to balance your whole body so that you can face situations in a calm and centred way. Strength increases our ability to handle life's ups and downs successfully. Practise this workout anytime you need strength.

1 The brain `1`

Finger walk the brain area using
the caterpillar movement.

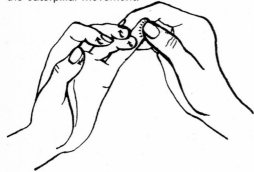

2 The pituitary gland `5`

Hook into this point, using your thumb.

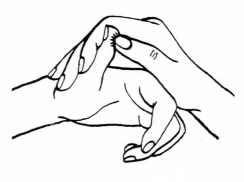

3 The thyroid gland `12`

Use your thumb to caterpillar walk the gland.

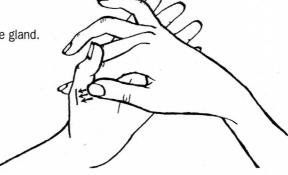

4 The lungs `13` and diaphragm `18`

Work this large area using the caterpillar movement
across your hands.

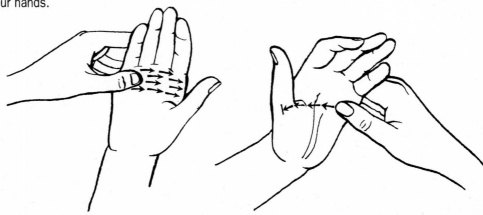

5 The adrenal glands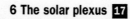

The adrenal glands are located near your kidneys; work them using the caterpillar walk.

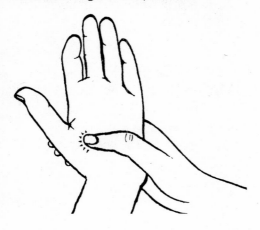

6 The solar plexus 17

Press your thumb into the solar plexus point, add pressure, then caterpillar walk over the point.

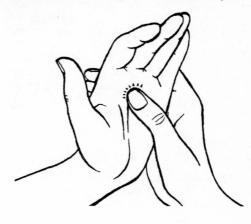

7 The kidneys 27

Work the bean-shaped kidney area with your thumb.

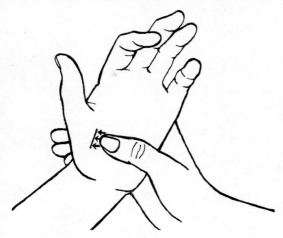

8 The spine 52, 53, 54, 56

Caterpillar walk down your spinal reflex points.

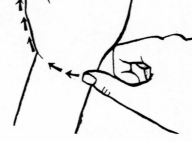

9 The sacro-ileac joint 55

Use the hook movement to work the sacro-ileac joint reflex, using gentle pressure.

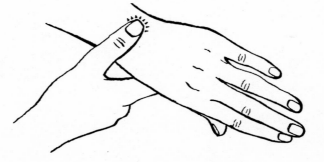

The Vitality Workout

TIME: 10 minutes, up to 3 times per week, on your hands. Practise the general relaxation techniques on pp 28-29 for a few minutes before and after this workout.

Work the following reflex areas on both hands:

1 The pituitary gland [5]
To help balance your hormones and make you feel good.

2 The heart and heart-related areas [16] and lungs [13]
To help boost your circulation and encourage you to breathe properly.

3 The solar plexus [17]
To help boost your energy by releasing nervous tension from your body.

4 The adrenal glands [26]
To help boost your adrenaline level to get your energies going.

5 The pancreas [25]
To help balance your blood sugar levels.

6 The small intestines [42]
To help speed up the digestive process and release toxins from your digestive system.

7 The spine [52], [53], [54], [56]
To help relax your whole body, stimulate and calm your nerves and improve your circulation.

8 The sacro-ileac joint [55]
To help relax your lower back.

For a complete guide to the numbered points refer to the easy reference charts on pp 115-119

COMPLAINT:
Dull complexion, tired eyes, lethargy.

CAUSE:
You may lose your vitality as a result of general illness in your body, a sluggish circulation and immune system, from suppressed and depressed emotions or from overactivity during the working day.

HOW REFLEXOLOGY HELPS:
Reflexology can help you by stimulating your whole body's energies and connecting you to your inner desires and inspirations. When you are inspired, your vitality increases. You have a *sparkle* in your eye, a joie de vivre that uplifts you and inspires everyone around you. You can practise this routine anytime during the day to help energize your whole body.

Self-Help for Energy and Vitality

1 The pituitary gland 5
Hook into your pituitary gland, using your thumb.

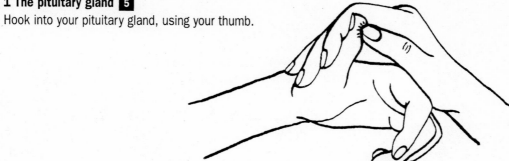

2 The heart and heart-related areas 16 and lungs 13
Work across the lungs area, using the caterpillar movement. Then work on the heart reflexes.

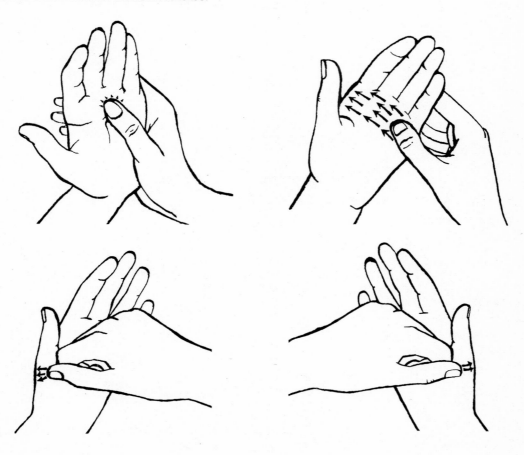

3 The solar plexus 17
Use your thumb to place pressure on this area, then release

4 The adrenal glands 26
Caterpillar walk over the adrenals.

5 The pancreas 27
Left hand only. Work into your pancreas with your thumb, using the caterpillar movement.

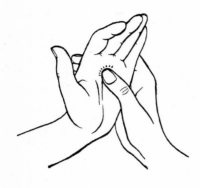

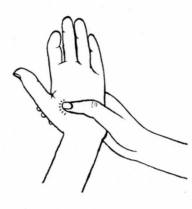

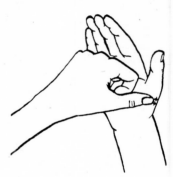

6 The small intestines 42
Work across your small intestines using the caterpillar walk.

7 The spine 52, 53, 54, 56
With your thumb, work down your hand from thumb to base, using the caterpillar movement

8 The sacro-ileac joint 55
Hook into this point gently, using your thumb.

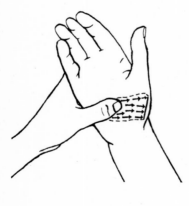

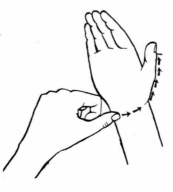

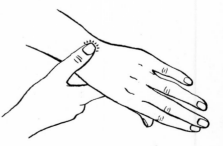

The Relaxation Workout (for healthy people)

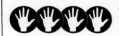 **TIME:** 20 minutes, up to 3 times per week, on both your feet. Practise the general relaxation techniques on pp 28-29 for a few minutes before and after this workout.

Work the following reflex areas on both feet:

1 The pituitary gland `5`
To help balance your hormones to keep you feeling happy and calm.

2 The chest, lungs `13` **and diaphragm** `18`
To help release tension from your breathing and so relax your body.

3 The solar plexus `17`
To help release tension from your whole nervous system.

4 The spine `52`, `53`, `54`, `56`
To help calm your whole body, and stimulate your circulation and nerve responses.

5 The sacro-ileac joint `55`
To help relax your lower back.

For a complete guide to the numbered points refer to the easy reference charts on pp 115-119

COMPLAINT:
You feel restless, nervous and tense.

CAUSE:
Tension in a healthy person can be caused by generally overdoing the good things in life or from too much excitement. Alternatively, you may feel generally tense because of noise (traffic, loud music, baby crying, etc.) or from a lack of exercise.

HOW REFLEXOLOGY HELPS:
Your reflexology workout can uplift and relax you. It helps to balance your whole body and allows tension to float away. You may like to practise it when you have nothing else to do in particular but to spoil yourself. Why not be completely self-indulgent? This workout can help keep you happy and feeling good all over. When you feel comfortable and relaxed, your inner beauty will shine through.

1 The pituitary gland `5`
Use your thumb to hook into the pituitary point.

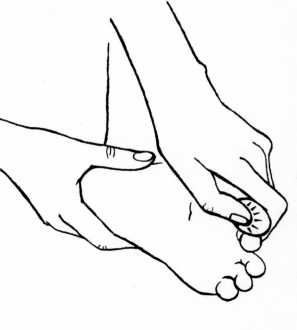

2 The chest, lungs 13 and diaphragm 18

Work across this area with your thumb, using the caterpillar walk.

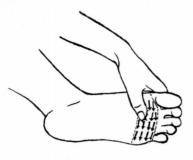
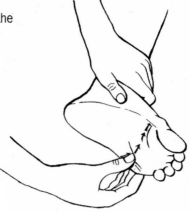

3 The solar plexus 17

Put pressure on this point with your thumb, then release.

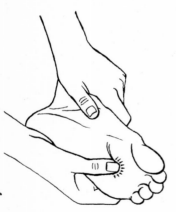

4 The spine 52, 53, 54, 56

Use your thumb to work down your spinal reflexes from the big toe area to the heel.

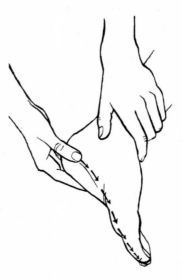

5 The sacro-ileac joint 55

Use hook movement with your thumb to work this reflex point gently.

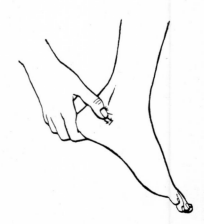

The Sex Workout

 TIME: 15 minutes, before sex, on your feet. Practise the general relaxation techniques on pp 28-29 before and after this workout.

Work the following reflex areas on both feet:

1 The brain 1
To help clear your mind of worries.

2 The pituitary 5
To help balance your hormones to make you feel good.

3 The neck and throat 7, 8
To help you express yourself and relax any tension in your neck area.

4 The heart and heart-related areas **16**
To help boost your circulation.

5 The breast 47, chest and lungs 13, and diaphragm 18
To help relax your breathing and increase your hormone production.

6 The solar plexus 17
To help relax your nerves and feel calm and centred.

7 The adrenal glands 26
To help balance your energy before sex.

8 The Fallopian tubes, seminal vesicles 46, uterus or prostate 45, ovaries or testes 44
To help balance your sexual areas (rather than stimulate them), in preparation for sex, which stimulates them enough!

9 The spine 52, 52, 54, 56
To help stimulate your nerves and circulation and help you relax.

10 The sacro-ileac joint 55
To help relax your lower back.

For a complete guide to the numbered points refer to the easy reference charts on pp 115-119

COMPLAINT:
Inability to obtain satisfaction from sex, either through full sexual intercourse or other stimulation.

CAUSE:
This can be due to you feeling pressure to perform, not feeling comfortable about yourself, not feeling safe with your partner or feeling insecure. You may have hang ups about your body because it's not 'perfect', you may be ill or not fit enough to enjoy satisfying sex, or may just be out of practice. You can also have a lot of sex but feel unsatisfied because your mind is elsewhere, perhaps because you aren't connecting with a sexual partner.

HOW REFLEXOLOGY HELPS:
Before sex, add a loving touch to your receptive body by practising reflexology on yourself or your partner. It is inviting and prepares you for intimacy by soothing and clearing your mind of worries and allowing you to unwind. In itself, reflexology doesn't turn you on (unless you have a sexual obsession with feet!) but it can help you to feel safe and

comfortable with your partner. It also encourages communication and creativity, which can help you express your preferences to your partner and be more adventurous. Reflexology between partners encourages an exchange of energies similar to those that take place during sex. Practising your sex reflexology workout together encourages you to be loving, affectionate and patient, and doesn't always need to lead to full sexual intercourse.

1 The brain 1
Use your finger to walk this area.

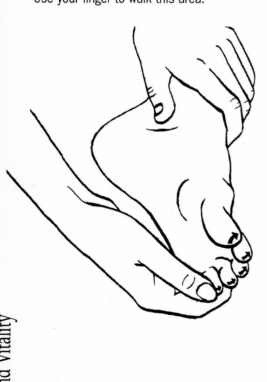

2 The pituitary gland 5
Use the hook movement with your thumb in the pituitary

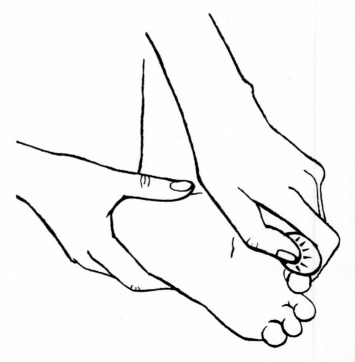

3 The throat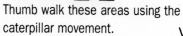

Thumb walk these areas using the
caterpillar movement.

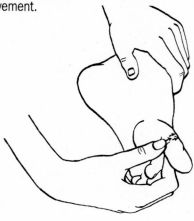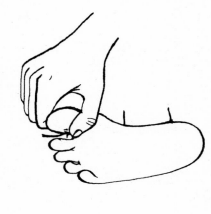

4 The heart and heart-related areas 16

Caterpillar walk these points, using your thumb.

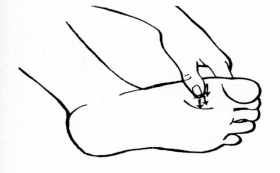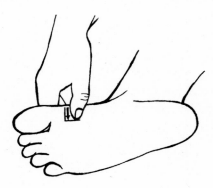

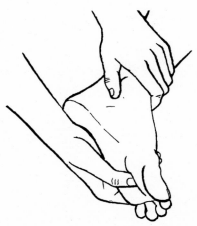

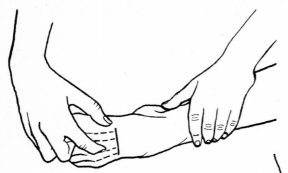

5 The breast **47**, chest and lungs **13**, and diaphragm **18**

Use your thumb to work across your chest, lung and diaphragm areas, using the caterpillar movement. Work your breast area gently, using the finger walk down your feet.

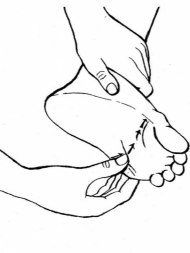

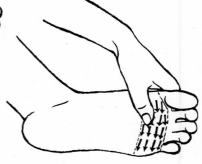

7 The adrenal glands **26**

Caterpillar walk this area with your thumb.

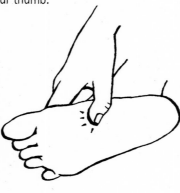

6 The solar plexus **17**

Use your thumb, adding pressure to this point, then release.

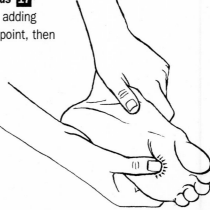

Self-Help for Energy and Vitality

8 The Fallopian tubes, seminal vesicles 46, uterus or prostate 45, ovaries or testes 44
Finger walk the Fallopian tubes and seminal vesicles 46 gently, using the caterpillar movement.

For the ovaries or testes 44, uterus or prostate 45, caterpillar walk the areas gently, using your finger or thumb.

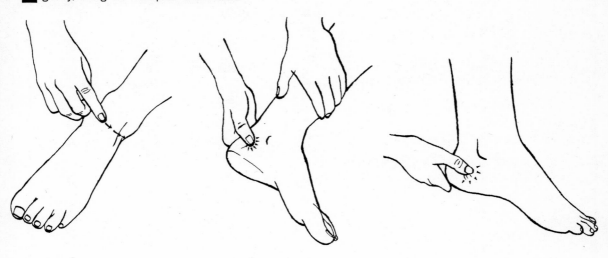

9 The spine 52, 53, 54, 56
Use your thumb to walk down your spine from the big toe area to the heel, using the caterpillar movement.

10 The sacro-ileac joint 55
Work this area using the hook technique.

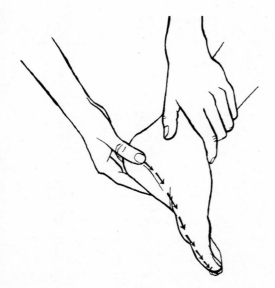

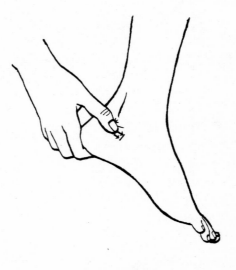

The Sex Workout

55

The Metabolism Workout

 TIME: 15 minutes, up to twice a week, on your hands. Practise the general relaxation techniques on pp 28-29 before and after this workout.

Work the following reflex areas on both your hands, except liver **19** and gall bladder **23**, right hand only; stomach **22** left hand only:

1 The thyroid gland 12
To help balance your metabolism.

2 The hypothalamus gland 4
To help balance and regulate your appetite.

3 The chest, lungs 13 and diaphragm 18
To help you breathe efficiently and so detoxify your body.

4 The stomach 22
To help stimulate your gastric juices, which aid digestion.

5 The pancreas 25
To help release pancreatic enzymes which help to break down food.

6 The liver 19
To help stimulate the formation of bile, to aid digestion.

7 The gall bladder 23
To help to release bile for digestion.

8 The adrenals 26
To help balance your energy and release hormones to balance your metabolism.

9 The kidneys 27
To help eliminate waste from your body and balance your water levels.

10 The intestines 30, 31, 33, 34, 37
To help eliminate waste and toxins from your body.

11 The solar plexus 17
To help calm your entire nervous system and help you feel relaxed.

For a complete guide to the numbered points refer to the easy reference charts on pp 115-119

COMPLAINT:
You may have a fast metabolism and be underweight or have a slow metabolism and be overweight. Both put a strain on your whole body, which you may not notice straightaway, but which after many years can lead to more serious illnesses.

CAUSE:
You may be overweight from eating too much fat, not taking enough exercise or your thyroid gland being under-efficient

(which means your metabolism functions more slowly). Women tend to put on weight more easily after the age of 30, during pregnancy and during the menopause, and men tend to gain weight around the age of 40. This is because your metabolism changes around these times. Being underweight is often the result of a fast metabolism – your thyroid gland functions very well. You may also lose weight if you 'live off your nerves', overexercise or simply don't eat enough.

Self-Help for Energy and Vitality

HOW REFLEXOLOGY HELPS:
Keeping your weight balanced is very important to health, and when your body feels loved and safe, it will find its own 'comfortable' weight and balance itself out. Reflexology can help in this by bringing balance and harmony to your whole body, including your metabolism, and helping you to accept the weight and shape you are. When you accept yourself you radiate inner happiness and joy.

1 The thyroid gland 12
Use your thumb to work into this area with the caterpillar movement.

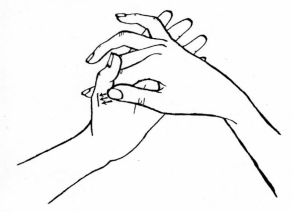

2 The hypothalamus gland 4
Hook into this point using your thumb or walk the gland with your thumb.

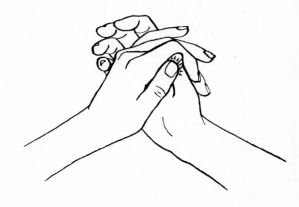

3 The chest, lungs 13 and diaphragm 18
Caterpillar walk across this whole area.

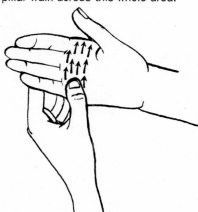

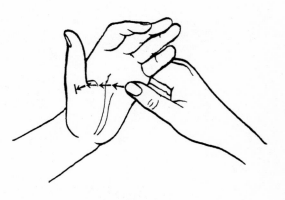

4 The stomach 22

Left hand only. Use your thumb to caterpillar walk across the stomach reflex area.

5 The pancreas 25

Use the caterpillar technique with your thumb to work the pancreas

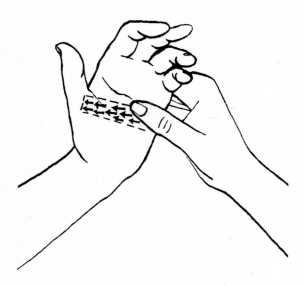

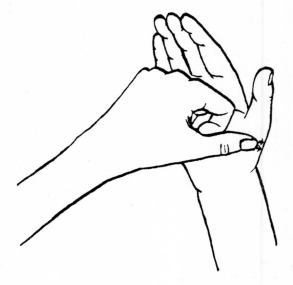

6 The liver 19

Right hand only. Work the whole area using the caterpillar movement with your thumb.

7 The gall bladder 23

Right hand only. Work into the area using your thumb in a caterpillar walk.

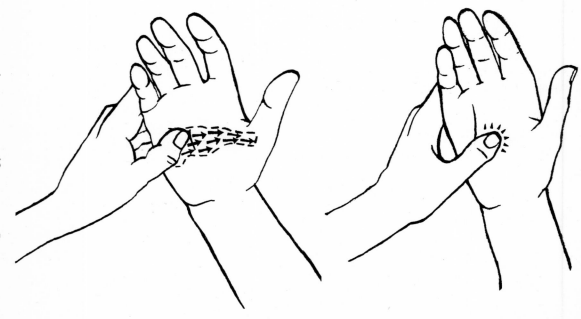

8 The adrenals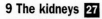
Caterpillar walk your adrenals using your thumb.

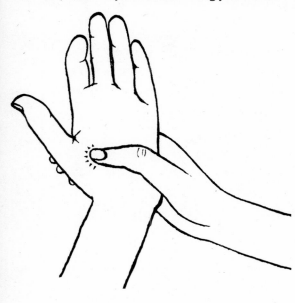

9 The kidneys 27
Work the bean-shaped organs using the caterpillar movement.

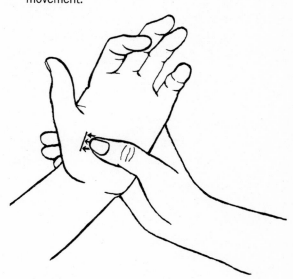

10 The intestines 30, 31, 33, 34, 37
Caterpillar walk across the area with your thumb.

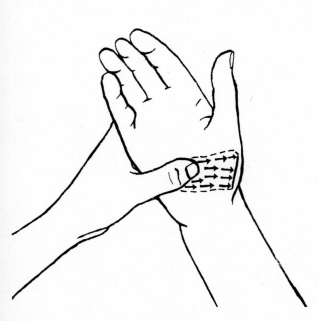

11 The solar plexus 17
Place pressure on this area with your thumb, then release.

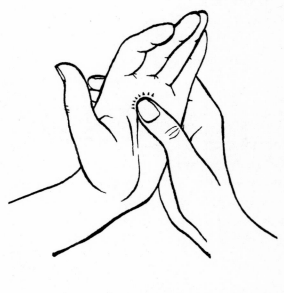

The Detoxification Workout

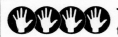 **TIME:** 20 minutes, twice per week, on your feet. Practise the general relaxation techniques on pp 28-29 before and after this workout.

Work the following reflex areas on both your feet, except liver **19**, ileocaecal valve **35**, right foot only; spleen **28**, left foot only.

1 The pituitary gland **5**
To help balance your emotions.

2 The lymph neck **7** , **8**
To help stimulate the detoxification process in that area.

3 The thymus gland **50**
To help produce T-lymphocytes, which help fight infection and detoxify your body.

4 The lymph breast **47** , **57**
To help cleanse and detoxify around your breasts.

5 The spleen **28**
To help detoxify your body and produce antibodies to fight infection.

6 The liver **19**
To help the formation of bile, for detoxification through digestion.

7 The adrenals **26**
To help produce anti-inflammatory hormones to fight infection.

8 The kidneys **27**
To help speed up the filtering of waste products through the digestive system.

9 The intestines **30** , **31** , **33** , **34** , **37**
To help stimulate the intestines to eliminate waste products from your body.

10 The ileocaecal valve (35)
To help prevent waste filtering back from your large to your small intestines.

11 The lymph groin (58)
To help detoxify your body in that area.

12 The solar plexus (17)
To help you to relax.

For a complete guide to the numbered points refer to the easy reference charts on pp 115-119

COMPLAINT:
You feel run down, you may have recurrent illnesses or infections which you are unable to throw off; you may have spots, skin rashes and other general aches and pains.

CAUSE:
Toxins build up in your body as a result of a poor diet (food additives, caffeine, etc.), stress, smoking and a lack of exercise. Environmental pollutants, such as car fumes, and industrial and chemical waste (particularly in large cities), also increase your absorption of toxins.

HOW REFLEXOLOGY HELPS:
Reflexology helps to detoxify your body by boosting your circulation and your immune system. So practising your self-help workout can help you be positive about your life and feel happy. One of the

best times to practise your detoxification workout is after you have fully recovered from an illness, when, by boosting your body's energies through reflexology, it can help prevent a recurrence and help bring your body back into harmony.

1 The pituitary gland 5
With your thumb, hook into this reflex point.

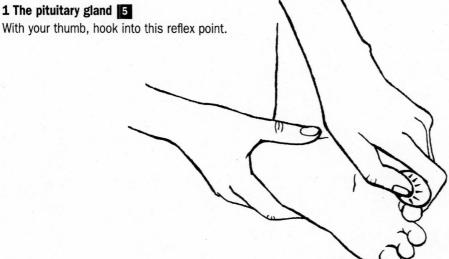

2 The lymph neck 7, 8
Use your finger or thumb in a caterpillar movement across this area.

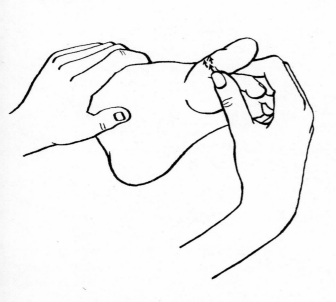

3 The thymus gland 50
Caterpillar walk the thymus gland, using your thumb.

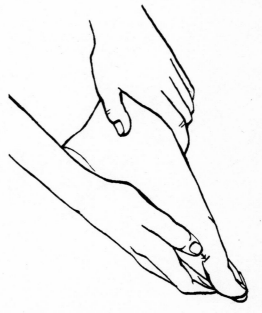

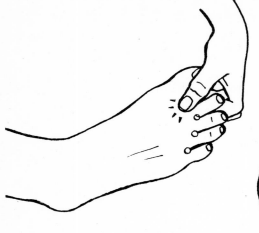

4 The lymph breast 47 , 57

For the breast areas, use your finger to work down and into the whole area using the caterpillar movement. The lymph breast points occur between each toe. Work each point between each toe.

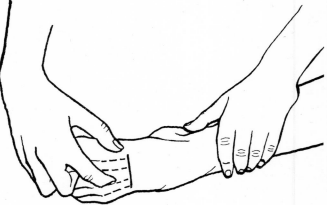

5 The spleen 28

Left foot only. Work your spleen with the caterpillar walk, using your thumb.

6 The liver 19

Right foot only. Work into and over your liver reflex using your thumb in a caterpillar movement.

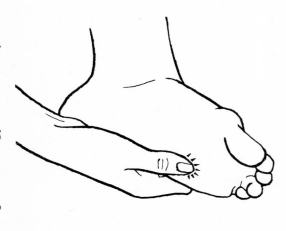

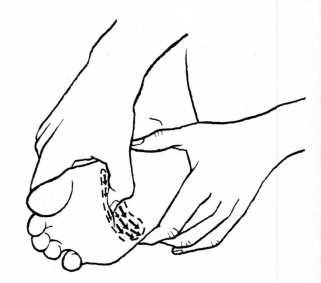

7 The adrenals 26

Thumb walk this area using the caterpillar technique.

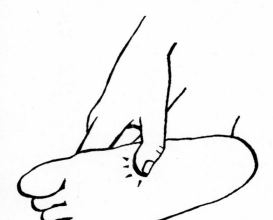

8 The kidneys 27

Caterpillar walk your bean-shaped kidney reflex areas using your thumb.

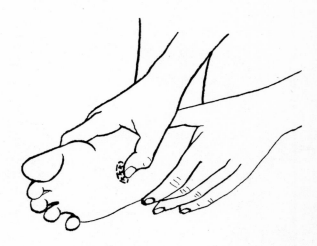

9 The intestines 30, 31, 33, 34, 37

Work across this large area using your thumb in a caterpillar walk.

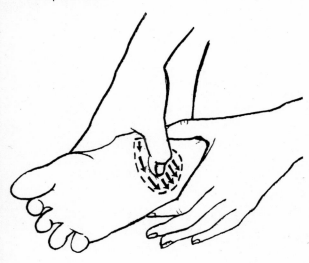

10 The ileocaecal valve 35

Thumb walk this area on your right foot only.

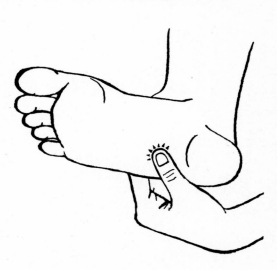

11 The lymph groin 58

Use your finger to walk this area using the caterpillar technique

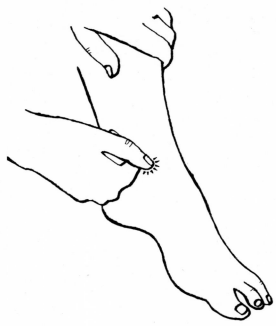

12 The solar plexus 17

Place pressure to this area using your thumb, then release.

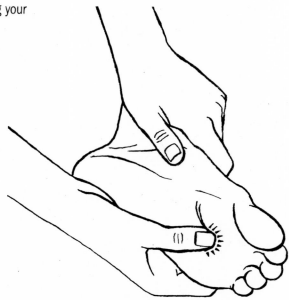

PART 3

Self-Help For Health

COMMON HEALTH COMPLAINTS

In this chapter are some self-help routines which, if followed carefully, can help you to manage some of the common complaints you may experience in your life – headaches, for example, which tend to occur when you least want them.

Practising reflexology on yourself encourages you to take responsibility for your health, to play an active role in your life instead of being a bystander. These routines are intended to help you get the most out of your life because when your body is balanced, you have more vitality and more to put into your life. This creates the potential for greater rewards, happiness and joy for yourself, and for others around you because when you are feeling happy it makes others happy too!

Start listening to your body and what it is trying to tell you. Listening to your body can help your life to flow more easily because by doing this you are learning to trust your instincts about your body's needs.

Self-help reflexology teaches you to rely on yourself, and to have fun and enjoyment with yourself too. Touch is very important – feeling safe to touch your own body can open you up to discovering your true self. Of course these simple techniques cannot replace visiting a professional reflexologist for a treatment – a professional reflexologist has often years of experience in knowing how to detect the whole picture of your health and has been fully trained. When you are ill you may prefer to visit a reflexologist

so that you can relax whilst you are worked on. Sometimes you don't have the energy to do it yourself. Being pampered by the healing touch of a reflexologist also makes you feel good. But in between treatments, these self-help routines are very useful.

These reflexology routines can help improve your health and regular practice can also help prevent recurring complaints such as sinusitis, headaches or constipation. Sometimes you may see an improvement in your health immediately. However, if you have suffered with a complaint for many years, it may take a while before you see any improvement or the complaint may even remain the same but you learn to manage it by practising your routines. You may even feel worse temporarily, whilst the toxins clear through your system. However, reflexology can help you to feel much happier in yourself so that you pay less attention to your complaints. Remember, however, you cannot use any of the reflexology routines to interpret or diagnose your health (not even professional reflexologists are able to do this unless they happen to be medical doctors as well).

These self-help routines are designed to work on your whole body and not just on your complaint, because reflexology uses the holistic approach. Therefore always practise the general relaxation techniques before and after working on any self-help routines, so that your whole body is worked. Read the 'Dos and Don'ts Checklist' on page 34 before working on yourself. If you are practising the self-help routines on someone else, ask them to do the same.

USING THE ROUTINES

Practise the general relaxation techniques on page 28 for a few minutes before and after working on any of the self-help routines. You will notice that each of these common complaints, listed in order from head to toe, indicates the amount of time to be spent working it and how often to practise it. Do stick to this.

Although each routine is illustrated as being practised on your hands or feet you can practise on either (but not both at once!) Simply note the numbers indicated with each reflex point and look them up on Jim Horan's maps of the feet and hands on pages 115-119.

Before you practise on your hands or feet, observe their looks. What temperature are they? What colour and texture are they? Do you have hard skin, corns, calluses or verrucaes and where are they in terms of your reflex areas of your body? Doing this check can give you a lot of clues as to which areas of your body are out of balance.

When practising your reflexology movements, find the pressure that feels comfortable for you. At times when your body feels sensitive (during your period, sickness, etc.), or if you generally have a sensitive body, you may need to work on your reflex points for a less amount of time than indicated. Remember never to overwork (hence overstimulate) your reflex points.

Also remember that when you practise your self-help reflexology routines you are looking to feel with your fingers or thumb areas of congestion or toxins, just underneath your skin. They may feel like tiny crystals, or gritty, sensitive or bruised, or you may feel a sharp pain when you work over them. This means that the corresponding areas of your body to those reflex points are out of balance at that moment in time. Each time you practise your reflex points may feel different. When you find an area of blockage, you need to spend more time working on those areas of your feet or hands. But again take care not to overwork your reflexes. Remember to practise only one self-help routine in any day and end your routine with a few minutes of deep breathing. It's best to avoid jogging or strenuous exercise after your reflexology to gain maximum benefits from your work.

If you are generally very healthy and fit you may like simply to practise the general relaxation techniques for 15 minutes, two to three times per week, rather than these routines to help maintain optimum health.

Headache

TIME: 10-15 minutes, three times per week, on both your hands. Practise the general relaxation techniques on pp 28-29 before and after this workout.

Work the following reflex areas on both hands except liver **19**, , ileocaecal valve **35**, right hand only; pancreas **25** left hand only:

1 The spine 52, 53, 54, 56
To help release general tension.

2 The brain and head 1
To help release pressure and fluid that have built up in and around the pain in your head.

3 The eyes 9
To help release tension and eye strain.

4 The sinuses 2
To help unblock the sinus area.

5 The pituitary gland 5
To help stimulate the endocrine system (balance the hormones).

6 The neck 7, 8
To help relax your neck muscles – tense muscles can bring on a headache.

7 The solar plexus 17
To help release stress and nervous tension.

8 The diaphragm 18
To help regulate your breathing, which may become shallow if you are tense.

9 The adrenals 26
To help reduce swelling and inflammation and also help to balance your emotions.

10 The liver 19
Right hand only. To help detoxify your blood, release glucose into your body, release bile and eliminate toxins

11 The stomach 22
Left hand only. To help stimulate the gastric juices to increase the productivity of the digestive system.

12 The pancreas 25
To balance blood sugar levels – a fluctuation in blood sugar levels may bring on a headache

13 The intestines 30, 33, 34, 37, 42
To help eliminate toxins from your body

14 The ileocaecal valve 35
Right hand only. To help prevent backflow of waste matter from your large to your small intestines and help the digestive system to flow freely.

For a complete guide to the numbered points refer to the easy reference charts on pp 115-119

COMPLAINT: When you get a headache you may experience a dull or sharp pain on the top or sides of your head (usually around the forehead). This pain can last from a few minutes to a few days, and may be persistent, or you may experience headaches on and off for years.

Right palm; repeat as left apart from liver **19**.

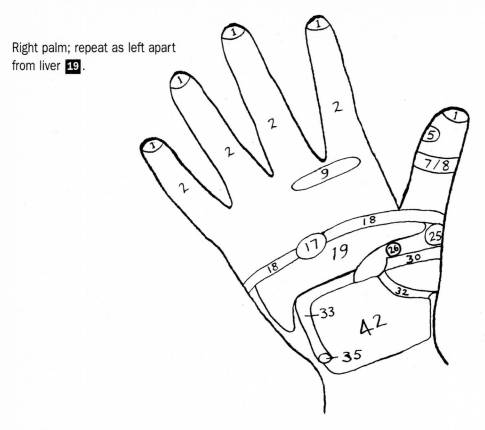

CAUSE:
Your headache can be a result of: misalignment of your spine, eye strain (especially if your need to wear glasses, are tired or have been working on a computer), shock, premenstrual tension, blood sugar imbalances (which in healthy people can be caused by eating irregularly), dehydration, blocked sinuses, constipation, sensitivity to daylight or bright lights, anger, being exposed to extremes in temperature, lack of exercise, poor posture, influenza, or from something more serious. As you might expect, headaches are very common and you may find yourself with one in many situations.

HOW REFLEXOLOGY HELPS:
Reflexology can help in many ways: by relaxing and oxygenating your body, by releasing toxins and stimulating your digestive system, and by helping to balance your whole body. It can also help you ward off illness – for example, if you know that you always get headaches before a period then you may like to start working on your self-help routine a few days before it's due to help prevent it or lessen its effects.

CAUTION:
This self-help routine is designed for a common/light headache. If you suffer from severe headaches or migraines and you are uncertain as to the cause, or there are other symptoms such as nausea, very high temperature or diarrhoea, it is important to seek medical advice.

Work left palm only.

25 22

Right top; repeat on other hand.

7/8

52

53

54

56

55

Blocked Sinuses

 TIME: Up to 10 minutes, twice per day, on both your hands. Practise the general relaxation techniques on pp 28-29 before and after this workout.

Work the following reflex areas on both hands:

1 The cervicals 52
To help release general tension from your face, head and neck and also boost your nerve supply to these areas.

2 The sinuses 2
To help release tension around this area.

3 The brain and head 1
To help release pressure and disperse the build up of fluid in your head and brain.

4 The pituitary 5
To help balance your hormones.

5 The eyes 9
To help release stress and tension around your eyes.

6 The lymph neck 7 , 8
To help stimulate the lymph and blood circulation to eliminate toxins.

7 The lymph breast 57
To help stimulate the lymph and blood circulation to eliminate toxins.

8 The bronchials 14
To help clear your bronchial tubes (part of your respiratory system) to help you breathe more easily.

9 The solar plexus 17
To help calm the whole nervous system.

10 The diaphragm 18
To help regulate your breathing, oxygenate your blood and help relax your muscles.

11 The adrenals 26
To help stimulate the production of hydrocortisone, which reduces any inflammation and helps you fight any infection.

For a complete guide to the numbered points refer to the easy reference charts on pp 115-119

COMPLAINT:
Pain around your eyes, nose and forehead, which can make it difficult to breathe; headaches, sneezing and a runny nose; dizziness. You may also feel tired and irritable and your throat or mouth may feel sore and dry.

CAUSE:
Stuffy rooms or atmospheres tend to provoke sinus pain; you may be in an office or home which isn't properly ventilated or outdoors in intense heat. General stress or allergies can bring on sinusitis and it can also accompany head colds. You may also develop sinusitis due to narrow nasal passages (from an accident or from the way you were born), which can play a part in recurrent attacks.

HOW REFLEXOLOGY HELPS:

Reflexology helps you relax and so releases tension in and around your head and sinus area. It helps stimulate your respiratory system so that you can breathe more easily. If you experience sinusitis attacks frequently, then practise reflexology regularly to help prevent it and help clear your sinus area in general.

Right top; repeat on other hand.

Right palm; repeat on other hand.

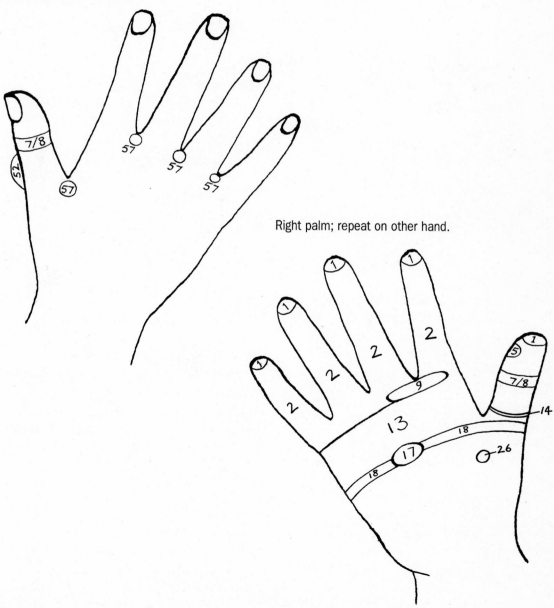

Eye Strain

 TIME: 10 minutes, three times per week, on your hands. Practise the general relaxation techniques on pp 28-29 before and after this workout.

Work the following reflex areas on both hands:

1 The brain and head `1`
To help you release tension and fluid build up in those areas.

2 The eyes `9`
To help relax and soothe the areas around your eyes.

3 The sinuses `2`
To help clear congestion and tension around your sinuses which may be adding to the tension around your eyes.

4 The cervicals `52`
To help increase the blood circulation and nerve activity to the whole of your head and neck area, and to relax you.

5 The solar plexus `17`
To help bring calm to your whole nervous system, and to help you relax.

6 The kidneys `27`
To help eliminate toxins and stale energy from around your body.

For a complete guide to the numbered points refer to the easy reference charts on pp 115-119

COMPLAINT:
With eye strain you may have a headache, be unable to focus fully, have bloodshot eyes and may screw up your eyes and not be able to tolerate strong artificial or natural light. Your eyeballs may feel heavy and you can feel dizzy or sick as a result of disorientation.

CAUSE:
Focusing on detailed work such as with a computer, sewing, doing your accounts, etc. for long periods of time, particularly in a poorly lit room. You may also have eye strain when you are out in bright sunshine, especially if you are sensitive to light, or if you need to wear glasses or need your current prescription for lenses changed, or if you are fatigued.

HOW REFLEXOLOGY HELPS:
Reflexology can help by encouraging relaxation and relieving stress and tension, particularly around your eyes, sinus, head and neck. When you are on your computer you can stop and practise this routine on your hands or when you are at home you can practise on your feet if you prefer. If you have eye strain from studying small print or reading a lot, remember to take breaks and structure your self-help routine into your day.

Left palm; repeat on other hand.

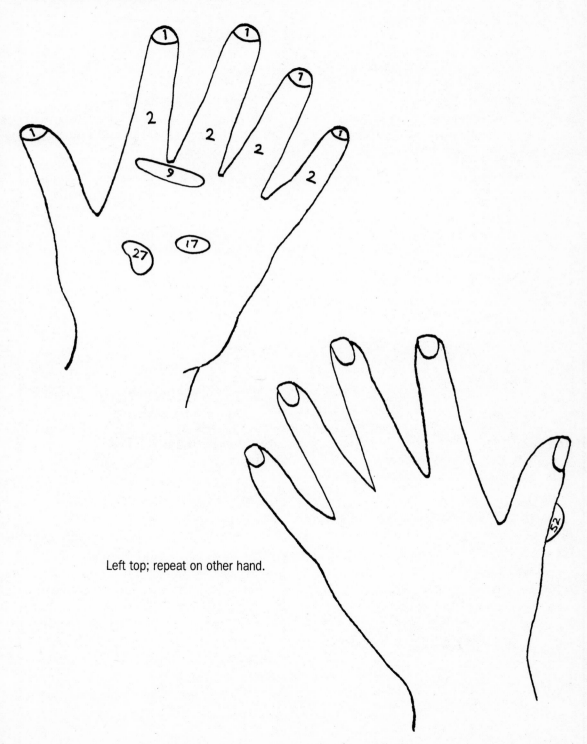

Left top; repeat on other hand.

Earache

 TIME: 15 minutes, up to three times per week, on your feet. Practise the general relaxation techniques on pp 28-29 before and after this workout.

Work the following reflex areas on both feet:

1 **The pituitary** 5
To help balance your hormones and keep you calm.

2 **The sinuses** 2
To help keep the area clear.

3 **The ears** 10
To help keep the circulation flowing.

4 **The eyes** 9
To help relax and relieve tension around your eyes.

5 **The cervicals** 52
To help provide blood supply to the nerves, which releases tension in your head and neck.

6 **The thymus gland** 50
To help encourage the production of T-lymphocytes, which help you to fight infection.

7 **The spleen** 28
Left foot only. To help the production of antibodies and detoxify your body.

8 **The lymph neck** 7 , 8
To help detoxify the area.

9 **The solar plexus** 17
To help calm and relax your nerves.

For a complete guide to the numbered points refer to the easy reference charts on pp 115-119

COMPLAINT:
A pain in one or both ears.

CAUSE:
The main cause of earache is a build up of fluid in the middle ear which has become infected. It can also be caused by exposure to strong winds, extremes in temperature, referral pain when your throat is inflamed, infection in your ears, loud noises or water being trapped behind earwax (from washing your hair or from swimming).

HOW REFLEXOLOGY HELPS:
Reflexology can help you by boosting your body's immune system to help fight any infection and stimulating your circulation to release toxins around your ears. When you have been skiing or out in cold winds, sit down and work on your feet as soon as you get indoors. If you are working on this routine for earache as part of a general infection, then keep warm and practise on yourself in bed or whilst resting in a chair. If you are prone to regular earache, make time for your self-help routine a few times a week to help keep you healthy. Enjoy looking after yourself.

Right sole; repeat on other foot.

Inside right foot.

2 2 2 2
5
7
2
9
8
10
17

52
50

Left sole only.

28

Toothache

 TIME: 10 minutes, twice per day, on your feet. Practise the general relaxation techniques on pp 28-29 before and after this workout.

Work the following reflex areas on both feet:

1 **The teeth and jaw** 43
To help release tension around your teeth and jaw, and boost your circulation in the area.

2 **The lymph neck and throat** 7 , 8
To help boost the immune system to fight any infection.

3 **The thymus gland** 50
To help encourage the production of

T-lymphocytes, which help boost the immune system.

4 **The sinuses** 2
To help relax your face and forehead area when you are feeling clogged up.

5 **The cervicals** 52
To help release tension in the whole of your head and neck area.

For a complete guide to the numbered points refer to the easy reference charts on pp 115-119

COMPLAINT:
Pain – a dull ache, niggling pain or intense sharp pain – in your teeth or gums.

CAUSE:
Toothache generally is caused by infection in your gums and from your teeth or gums decaying. You may also get it when you drink hot or cold drinks, or if you are out in extreme temperatures.

HOW REFLEXOLOGY HELPS:
Reflexology can help you by fighting any infection around your teeth, and by relaxing the nerves in your mouth and face. It is also useful in helping calm your whole body, because when you have toothache you tense up and this adds to the problem. Practising the day before or the day after visiting your dentist for treatment can help speed up your body's natural healing powers. Make sure you use a light pressure because your gums and teeth will be very sensitive.

Right sole; repeat on other foot.

Inside right foot; repeat on other foot.

2 2 2 2 7
8

52
50

43

Right foot top;
repeat on other foot.

The Common Cold

TIME: 15 minutes, up to three times per week, on your hands. Practise the general relaxation techniques on pp 28-29 before and after this workout.

Work the following reflex areas on both hands except spleen **28**, left hand only:

1 The brain and head **1**
To help release pressure from the cold in your head.

2 The eyes **9**
To help relax your eyes.

3 The ears **10**
To help stimulate your circulation to release blockages around your ears.

4 The lymph neck and throat **7**, **8**
To help you fight any infection.

5 The pituitary **5**
To helps stimulate and balance your hormones.

6 The chest and lung **13**
To help boost your circulation, help you breathe more easily and release tension.

7 The thymus **50**
To help you fight any infection.

8 The bronchials **14**
To help you to breathe more easily.

9 The thyroid gland **12**
To help keep your metabolism balanced.

10 The solar plexus **17**
To help calm you down and keep you calm.

11 The diaphragm **18**
To help oxygenate and detoxify your body.

12 The cervicals **52**
To help increase the blood supply to your nerves and relax your whole head and neck area.

13 The spleen **28**
Left hand only. To help you fight any infection.

14 The adrenal glands **26**
To help keep your emotions balanced.

15 The lymph chest and breast **47**, **57**
To help detoxify your body.

For a complete guide to the numbered points refer to the easy reference charts on pp 115-119

COMPLAINT:
You sneeze frequently and have a runny nose. You may also feel shivery and have a headache.

CAUSE:
Generally you catch a cold from someone you have come into contact with, but your chances are increased by getting wet, damp and cold. When you are run down or if you have not recovered properly from another illness you can catch colds easily and you may even experience recurrent colds.

HOW REFLEXOLOGY HELPS:
Reflexology helps by boosting your circulation and your lymphatics to help detoxify your body, clear any mucus from your head and chest, and generally relax.

Left palm; repeat on other hand
except spleen 28.

Left top; repeat on other hand.

The Common Cold

81

Hiccoughs

 TIME: 5-10 minutes, when you have hiccoughs, on your hands. Practise the general relaxation techniques on pp 28-29 before and after this workout.

Work the following reflex areas on both hands:

1 **The solar plexus** 17
   To help calm your whole nervous system.

2 **The diaphragm** 18
   To help encourage you to breathe deeply and relax your diaphragm.

3 **The pituitary** 5

To help calm your emotions.

4 **The chest and lungs** 13
   To help you to breathe deeply and release tension.

5 **The bronchials** 14
   To help clear your bronchial tubes so that you can breathe more easily.

For a complete guide to the numbered points refer to the easy reference charts on pp 115-119

COMPLAINT:
Loud involuntary 'hic' sounds; hiccoughs can also give you severe pain around your ribcage.

CAUSE:
Hiccoughs are caused by involuntary spasm from your diaphragm, which results in not enough oxygen entering your body. You get hiccoughs when you are not breathing properly, when you are trying to do two things at once – talk and eat, for example – or when you are drinking or eating too quickly.

HOW REFLEXOLOGY HELPS:
You can find yourself with hiccoughs in almost any situation and may feel embarrassed by them in a public place. Stop. Practise your self-help reflexology routine. This can help you to stay calm and help your body to return to its natural rhythm of breathing by opening up your ribcage and allowing more oxygen in, and by calming your nerves.

Right palm; repeat on other hand

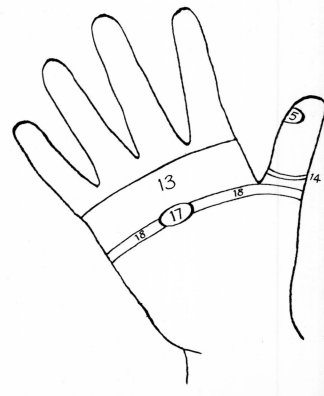

Sore Throat

TIME: 15 minutes, up to three times per week, on your hands. Practise the general relaxation techniques on pp 28-29 before and after this workout.

Work the following reflex areas on both hands:

1 The sinuses `2`
To help clear your sinus area and release tension.

2 The head `1`
To help relax the whole of your head.

3 The lymph neck and throat `7`, `8`
To help you release toxins and to fight any infection.

4 The thymus `50`
To help maintain immunity to disease and fight infection.

5 The adrenal glands `26`
To help reduce swelling or inflammation in your throat.

6 The cervicals `52`
To help you release tension in the whole of your neck and head and boost your circulation.

For a complete guide to the numbered points refer to the easy reference charts on pp 115-119

COMPLAINT:
You may suffer pain and feel that your throat is raw. Sometimes your throat may be so inflamed that it is difficult for you to swallow food or drink.

CAUSE:
You can find yourself with a sore throat from a viral or bacterial infection, from straining your voice by singing, talking too much or shouting, or from an allergy or exposure to smoky, dry or hot air.

HOW REFLEXOLOGY HELPS:
Reflexology can help you reduce any inflammation around your throat and boost your immune system to fight infection.

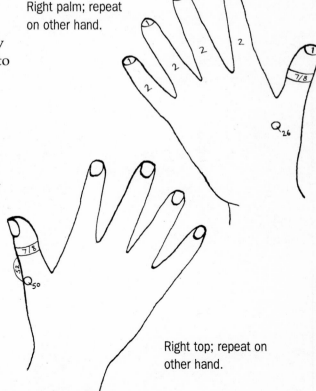

Right palm; repeat on other hand.

Right top; repeat on other hand.

Sore Throat

Cough

Work the following reflex areas on both feet:

1 The throat 7 , 8
To help relax your throat muscles – coughing causes you to tense up and when you relax sometimes your cough eases up.

2 The thymus 50
To help boost your immune system by encouraging production of T-lymphocytes to help fight infection.

3 The diaphragm 18
To help regulate your breathing, and oxygenate your blood.

4 The lungs 13
To help release tension, and help you breathe more easily.

5 The solar plexus 17
To help calm your nerves and relax you.

6 The adrenal glands 26
To help reduce swelling around your throat by encouraging the production of hydrocortisone.

For a complete guide to the numbered points refer to the easy reference charts on pp 115-119

COMPLAINT:
A loud or irritating cough from your throat, either dry or with mucus.

CAUSE:
Coughing is a reflex action caused by your lungs clearing out any irritation. It can be set off by allergies: dust, pollution, perfumes, cats and dogs, etc. A cough can also occur when you are fighting an infection in the throat or lungs or from catarrh clearing the lungs. You may have a dry cough from thirst or because of a psychological reason, for instance, when you are feeling nervous or scared you may get a fit of coughing.

HOW REFLEXOLOGY HELPS:
Reflexology helps relax your whole body and fight any infection in and around your throat and lungs. Coughing can occur at any time, so it may be helpful to memorize this self-help routine.

Self-Help For Health

Right sole; repeat on other foot.

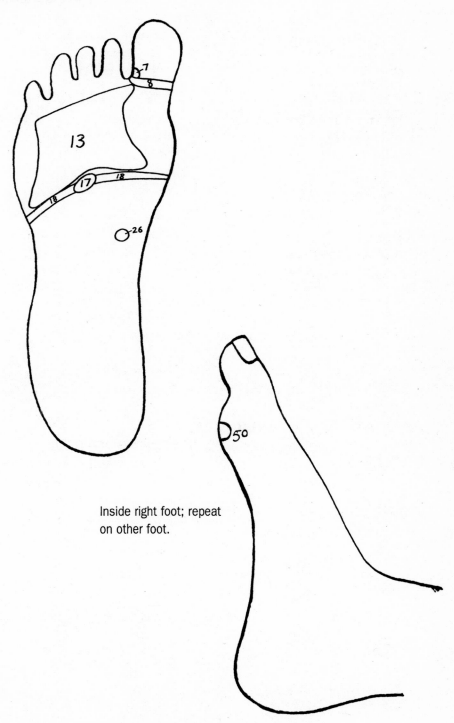

Inside right foot; repeat
on other foot.

Hangover

TIME: 20 minutes, at the onset of your hangover, on your feet. Practise the general relaxation techniques on pp 28-29 before and after this workout.

Work the following reflex areas on both feet except liver **19**, right foot only:

1 **The spine** **52**, **53**, **54**, **56**
To help you relax your whole body.

2 **The thyroid gland** **12**
To help balance your metabolism.

3 **The solar plexus** **17**
To help calm your whole nervous system.

4 **The kidneys** **27**
To help eliminate toxins from your body and keep your water levels balanced.

5 **The adrenals** **26**
To help balance your potassium, salt and water levels, blood sugar levels and blood pressure.

6. **The liver** **19**
Right foot only. To help detoxify your blood and form bile to help eliminate toxins from the digestive system.

7. **The sacro-ileac joint** **55**
To help relax the lower back.

For a complete guide to the numbered points refer to the easy reference charts on pp 115-119

COMPLAINT:
You may experience any of the following with a hangover: a cloudy head, disorientation, an inability to concentrate, extreme tiredness, dehydration, nausea and a furry tongue.

CAUSE:
Low blood sugar is a major factor with a hangover. You can find yourself with a hangover when you have consumed too much alcohol or from drinking very little but on an empty stomach.

HOW REFLEXOLOGY HELPS:
Reflexology helps by balancing your body's water levels, eliminating toxins and calming your nervous system. It is best to practise your self-help routine as soon as you feel a hangover coming on.

Self-Help For Health

Right sole; repeat on other foot except liver **19**.

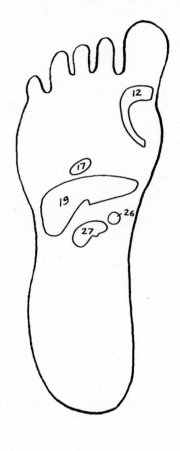

Inside right foot; repeat on other foot.

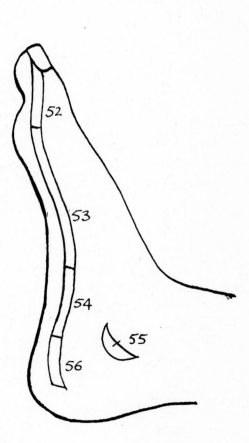

Tiredness

 TIME: 15 minutes, three to four times per week, on your feet Practise the general relaxation techniques on pp 28-29 before and after this workout.

Work the following reflex areas on both feet:

1 **The thyroid gland** 12
To help balance your metabolism.

2 **The solar plexus** 17
To help calm your nerves.

3 **The diaphragm** 18
To help relax and deepen your breathing and oxygenate your blood. When you are tired often your breathing becomes irregular and shallow.

4 **The pancreas** 25
Left foot only. To help balance your blood sugar levels.

5 **The adrenals** 26
To help produce adrenaline, balance blood pressure and stabilize blood sugar levels.

6 **The spine** 52, 53, 54, 56
To help stimulate your whole body.

7. **The sacro-ileac joint** 55
To help relax the lower back.

For a complete guide to the numbered points refer to the easy reference charts on pp 115-119

COMPLAINT:
Your body feels heavy, as though you are dragging it around. You have difficulty staying awake and alert.

CAUSE:
If you are suffering from depression and anxiety, a continual lack of sleep or too much sleep, a lack of exercise or too much exercise, stress or trauma, you can feel tired. You may be constantly tired from overwork, especially if you have to look after babies or young children, or if you are under a lot of pressure at work with deadlines to meet or a difficult boss. A lack of motivation or stimulation in your lifestyle can make you feel generally tired but unable to fall asleep

HOW REFLEXOLOGY HELPS:
Reflexology can really help to pick you up and at the same time relax you from the stresses and strains of daily life. You can practise your self-help routine at home or at work, sitting in a chair or lying down. Ideally, practise for the full 15 minutes, but if you are too tired then start off with a few minutes and do more when you feel you can.

Left sole; repeat on other foot except pancreas **25**.

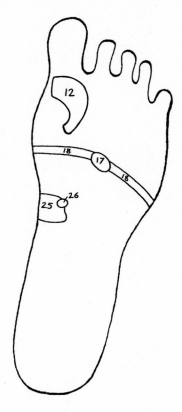

Right inside foot; repeat on
other foot.

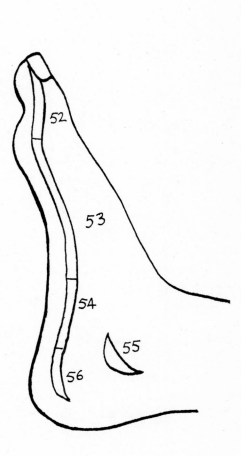

Sleeplessness

TIME: 15 minutes, before bedtime or when you wake in the night, on your hands or feet. Practise the general relaxation techniques on pp 28-29 before and after this workout.

Work the following reflex areas on both hands:

1 The head `1`
To help calm your mind.

2 The solar plexus `17`
To help soothe your nerves.

3 The diaphragm `18`
To help you relax and deepen your breathing.

4 The heart and heart-related areas `16`
To help stabilize your breathing and relaxes the heart muscle.

For a complete guide to the numbered points refer to the easy reference charts on pp 115-119

COMPLAINT:
Sleeplessness is the inability to go to sleep, but you may also find your sleep interrupted, or wake up frequently throughout the night.

CAUSE:
Sleeplessness can be due to worries, trauma, excitement or restlessness caused by general illness in your body. It may be the result of overtiredness or of eating too much before your bedtime. Alternatively, if you are very hungry low blood sugar can also keep you awake. Sleeplessness can be a particular problem for those who work shifts or fly a lot.

HOW REFLEXOLOGY HELPS:
Reflexology can help you to relax your mind, body and spirit. You can practise in bed or in a chair; people often report falling asleep before finishing this routine!

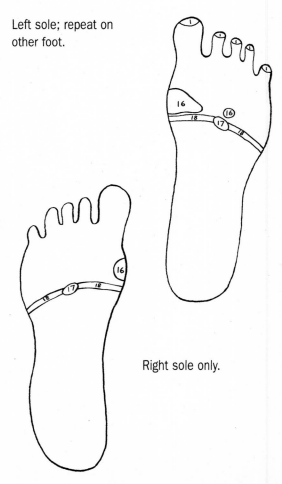

Left sole; repeat on other foot.

Right sole only.

Poor Circulation

TIME: 10 minutes, up to 3 times per week, on your hands. Practise the general relaxation techniques on pp 28-29 for a few minutes before and after this workout.

Work the following reflex areas on both hands:

1 **The lymph 7, 49, 57, 58**
To help detoxify your body.

2 **The heart and heart-related areas 16**
To help increase the blood supply to your body to boost your circulation.

3 **The spine 52, 53, 54, 56**
To help stimulate the blood circulation and nerves.

For a complete guide to the numbered points refer to the easy reference charts on pp 115-119

COMPLAINT

When you have a weak circulation you may feel constantly cold, especially in your hands and feet.

CAUSE

This is caused by your blood not pumping around your body efficiently. Your arteries may be clogged (atherosclerosis) or go into spasm. A poor circulation can be hereditary or a result of shock, being underweight, not eating enough food or lack of exercise

HOW REFLEXOLOGY HELPS

Reflexology helps you get your whole circulation moving. This routine can be particularly beneficial when you are out in the cold. When you first practise it, sit down and concentrate on working your reflex points correctly, but when you are used to the routine, you can do it on the move.

Left palm only.

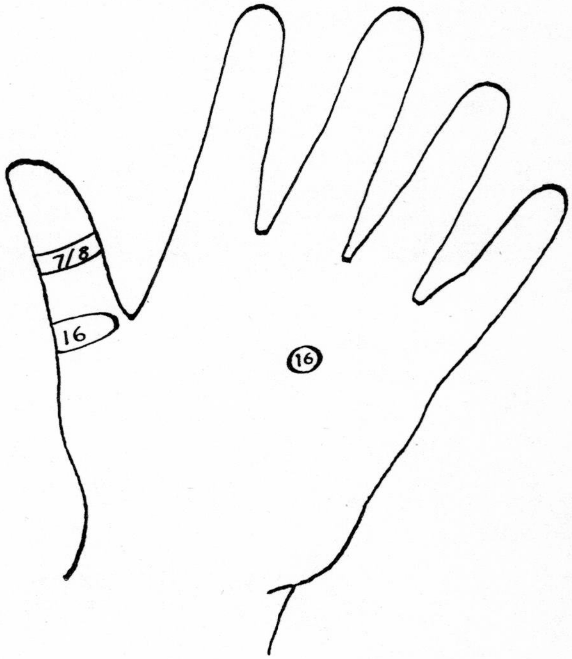

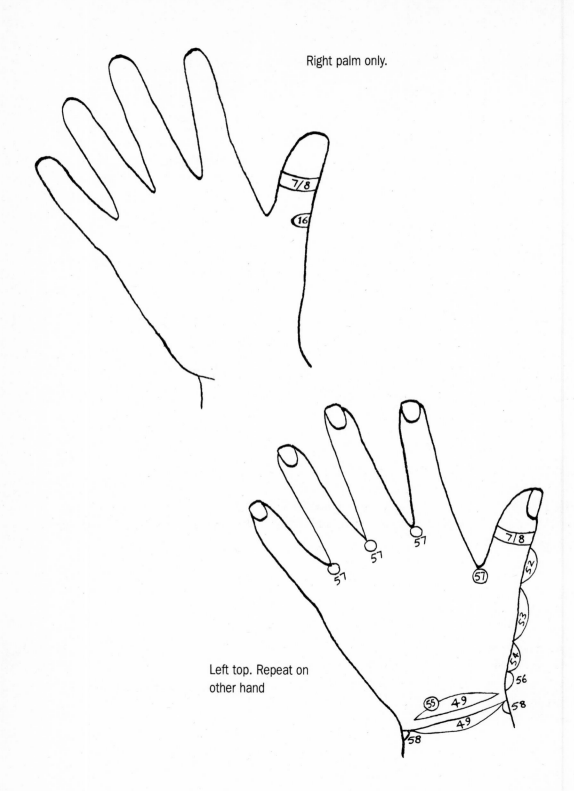

Right palm only.

7/8

16

57

57

57

57

7/8

52

53

54

56

55 4·9

58

4·9

58

Left top. Repeat on
other hand

Stress

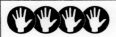 **TIME:** 20 minutes, up to four times per week, on your feet. Practise the general relaxation techniques on pp 28-29 for a few minutes before and after this workout.

Work the following reflex areas on both feet:

1 **The adrenal glands** 26
To help calm your emotions.

2 **The solar plexus** 17
To help calm your nerves.

3 **The spine pituitary** 5
To help balance your emotions.

4 **The chest and lungs** 13
To help relax your breathing.

5 **The brain and head** 1
To help still your mind from worrying about problems.

6 **The heart and related areas** 16
To help release tension in your heart muscle and boost the circulation of blood around your body.

7 **The spine** 52, 54, 56
To help relax your whole body.

For a complete guide to the numbered points refer to the easy reference charts on pp 115-119

COMPLAINT

Nervous tension puts pressure on all the systems of your body, often resulting in illness. As already mentioned, a little stress is helpful, but if you have constant stress in your life you are more likely to get ill and less likely to throw the illness off easily.

CAUSE

Stress can be a result of one or a combination of circumstances in your life: problems with your relationships, changing your career, health problems, difficult children or problems in your environment (pollution, noise, food additives, etc.).

HOW REFLEXOLOGY HELPS

Reflexology can help you to face the problems which are causing you stress. It can help to relax you, encourage you to communicate your problems to others (a problem shared is a problem halved) and can help you take responsibility for your life. Practise your self-help routine when you have time to set aside 20 minutes without outside interruptions, preferably at home. However, if sitting down for 20 minutes is going to cause you stress in itself, then practise for a shorter time. As you start to enjoy it and feel more relaxed you can give yourself the full 20 minutes.

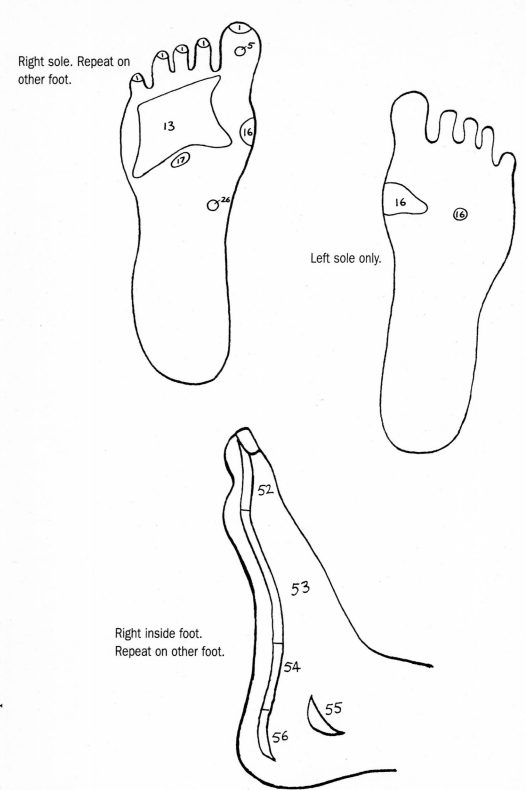

Right sole. Repeat on
other foot.

Left sole only.

Right inside foot.
Repeat on other foot.

Travel Stress

Work the following reflex areas on both hands:

1 **The adrenal glands** 26
   To help calm you.

2 **The solar plexus** 17
   To help calm your entire nervous system and relax your body.

3 **The pituitary gland** 5
   To help keep your hormones balanced.

4 **The pineal gland** 4
   To help you to adjust to any hormonal changes within your body,
   either from jet lag or from adjusting to other time zones.

5 **The inner ear** 10
   To help maintain your equilibrium and keeps you balanced.

6 **The spine** 52, 53, 54, 56
   To help relax your entire body, calm your nerves and stimulate your circulation.

7. **The sacro-ileac joint** 55
   To help relax the lower back.

For a complete guide to the numbered points refer to the easy reference charts on pp 115-119

COMPLAINT:
During your travels you may feel tired, lethargic, anxious, nervous and restless. You may be unable to sleep even when you try, may feel travel sick or become dehydrated.

CAUSE:
Travel stress can occur from a change in your metabolism, from jet lag when you cross different time zones, from the movement of a vehicle or from feeling anxious or excited about your journey. You may also feel angry, confused, frustrated and disorientated by cancellations or delays in your schedule.

HOW REFLEXOLOGY HELPS:
Practising your self-help routine before your journey helps you relax. Reflexology
during your journey can ward off sickness and help keep you balanced and calm. Working on yourself after your journey can help to bring harmony back to your whole body and help you to settle in to your environment.

Left palm; repeat on other side.

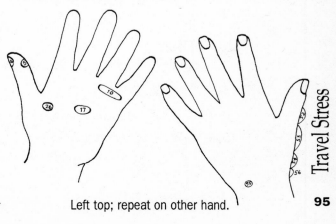

Left top; repeat on other hand.

Backache

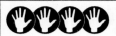

TIME: 20 minutes, up to three times per week, on your feet. Practise the general relaxation techniques on pp 28-29 before and after this workout.

Work the following reflex areas on both feet:

1 The solar plexus `17`
To help calm your whole body.

2 The diaphragm `18`
To help oxygenate your body and relax your breathing.

3 The shoulder and arm `15`
To help relax these areas.

4 The neck `7`, `8`
To help relax your whole neck area.

5 The sciatic nerve `41`
To help improve your circulation and relax any tension in the nerve.

6 The hip and knee `48`
To help relax you and release tension in these areas.

7 The spine `52`, `53`, `54`, `56`
To help relax your body and stimulate your circulation so that fresh oxygen is supplied to areas of tension.

8. The sacro-ileac joint `55`
To help relax the lower back.

For a complete guide to the numbered points refer to the easy reference charts on pp 115-119

COMPLAINT
The ache or pain may be in a general area like the upper, lower or middle back, or in a specific area like the shoulders or the neck.

CAUSE:
Back pain is one of the most common symptoms of disease in the world today. It may occur for many reasons: poor posture, an accident, lifting heavy objects, trauma, premenstrual tension, influenza or some other disease. There has been some medical research to suggest that backache and back injury are more likely to occur when your blood sugar levels are low or when you are very tense.

HOW REFLEXOLOGY HELPS:
Reflexology can help you manage back pain and act as a preventative by keeping your muscles relaxed and supple. It promotes oxgenation of the areas where toxins have built up causing stiffness and pain. Make sure you are sitting in a comfortable, firm chair and your spine is upright when you work on this routine.

CAUTION:
This self-help routine is designed for people with aches rather than chronic or serious back problems. Always ask your doctor to diagnose any back pain.

Self-Help For Health

96

Right sole; repeat on other foot.

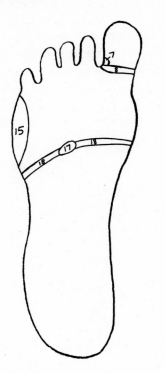

Inside right foot; repeat on other foot.

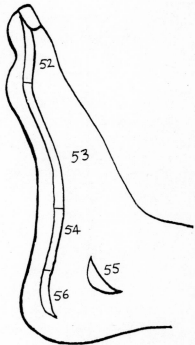

Outside right foot; repeat on other side.

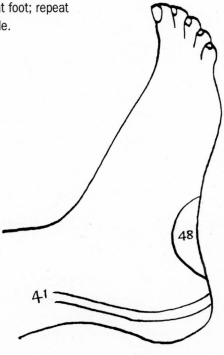

Premenstrual Tension
(BLOATING, BACKACHE)

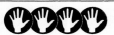 **TIME:** 20 minutes, only once per day, three times during the week before menstruation and/or at the end of menstruation, on your feet. Practise the general relaxation techniques on pp 28-29 before and after this workout.

Work the following reflex areas on both feet except liver **19**, right foot only; spleen **28** left foot only:

1 The solar plexus 17
To help calm your nervous system.

2 The kidneys 27
To help eliminate toxins from your body.

3 The liver 19
Right foot only. To help detoxify your blood and balance your water levels.

4 The thyroid gland 12
To help balance your energy levels, which can be low during your period.

5 The parathyroid 12
To help maintain your phosphorus and calcium levels.

6 The adrenal glands 26
To help maintain your mineral levels and balance your body's energy.

7 The lymph breast 47, 57
To help reduce swelling in the breast and boost your lymph circulation.

8 The spleen 28
Left foot only. To help detoxify your body.

9 The ovaries 44
To help formulate the hormones oestrogen and progesterone.

10 The uterus 45
To help keep your circulation moving to allow blood flow.

11 The Fallopian tubes 46
To help release tension and keep the area clear.

12 The lumber spine 54
To help relax the muscles in your lower back.

For a complete guide to the numbered points refer to the easy reference charts on pp 115-119

COMPLAINT:
Premenstrual tension can produce lower backache, cramps and/or abdominal bloating .

CAUSE:
This type of PMT is caused by fluid retention, and cramps in the pelvic area, from two weeks to a day before menstruation. You may also experience symptoms during your period although most women find PMT eases off after the first few days.

HOW REFLEXOLOGY HELPS:
If you practise your self-help routine before your period it can help to boost your circulation, detoxify your body and

stimulate your endocrine system, which can help reduce the severity of your symptoms. This routine also the menstrual flow to begin (as a result of the stimulation to your reproductive area and through general relaxation), and if you practise reflexology towards the end of your period it can help bring it to an end.

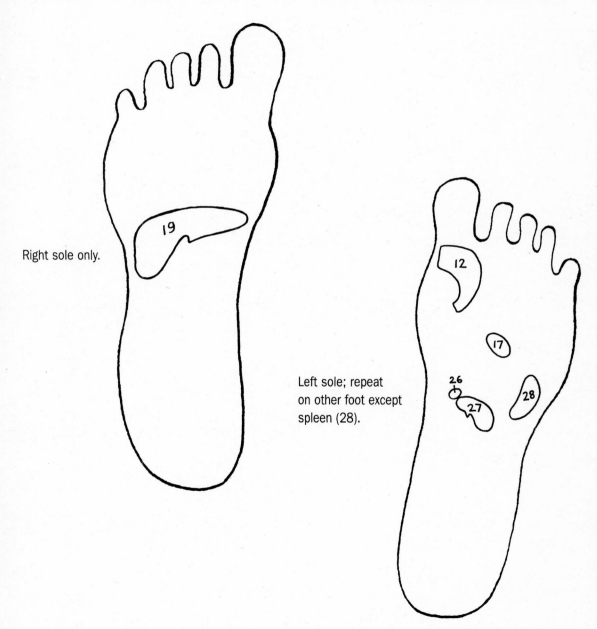

Right sole only.

Left sole; repeat on other foot except spleen (28).

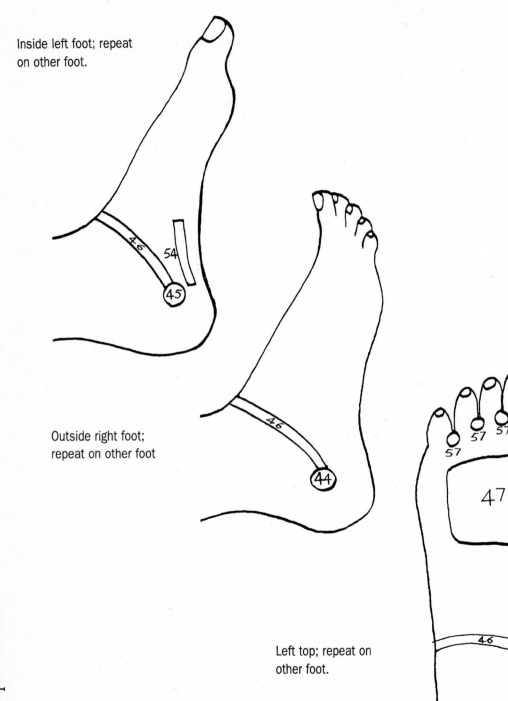

Inside left foot; repeat
on other foot.

Outside right foot;
repeat on other foot

Left top; repeat on
other foot.

Premenstrual Tension
(HEADACHES, EMOTIONAL)

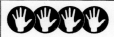 **TIME:** 20 minutes, only once per day, three times during the week before menstruation, on your hands. Practise the general relaxation techniques on pp 28-29 before and after this workout.

Work the following reflex areas on both hands:

1 **The pituitary** `5`
To help boost all your endocrine organs which helps to keep your mood and your hormones balanced.

2 **The sinuses** `2`
To help release tension from the sinuses.

3 **The brain and head** `1`
To help you still your mind and release tension and irritability.

4 **The neck** `7`, `8`
To help you relax your neck muscles.

5 **The eyes** `9`
To help release tension from around your eyes.

6 **The diaphragm** `18`
To help the body to breathe and oxygenate the blood.

7 **The solar plexus** `17`
To help calm your nerves.

8 **The spine** `52`, `53`, `54`, `56`
To help improve your circulation, and help release muscular tension around your spine.

9. **The sacro-ileac joint** `55`
To help relax the lower back.

For a complete guide to the numbered points refer to the easy reference charts on pp 115-119

COMPLAINT:
Premenstrual tension can result in your feeling very emotional – weepy, angry, aggressive, impatient, irrational and sometimes violent. You may also feel confused and clumsy and be prone to headaches.

CAUSE:
Around the time of menstruation your hormone levels change which can create emotional imbalance and tension.

HOW REFLEXOLOGY HELPS:
Reflexology helps before and during your period by relaxing your whole body and works on your endocrine system to help balance your body. It's best to practise your routine first thing in the morning or in the evening. If your PMT develops into a form of depression each month, your mood swings become extreme or you get migraines, you should discuss this with your doctor.

Right top; repeat
on other hand.

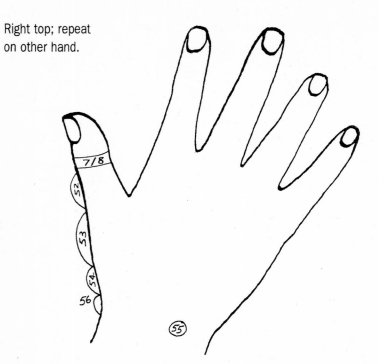

Right palm; repeat
on other hand.

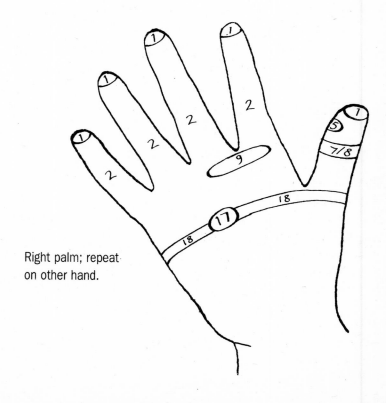

Constipation

 TIME: 15 minutes, up to three times per week, on your feet. Practise the general relaxation techniques on pp 28-29 before and after this workout.

Work the following reflex areas on both feet except liver **19**, ileocaecal valve **35**, gall bladder **23**, right foot only:

1 **The solar plexus** **17**
To help increase nerve activity and release tension.

2 **The lumber spine** **54**
To release tension in your lower back.

3 **The intestines** **30**, **31**, **33**, **34**, **37**, **42**
To help free up the intestines by releasing tension and boosting your circulation.

4 **The adrenal glands** **26**
To help release adrenaline to boost your energy levels and get things moving.

5 **The liver** **19**
Right foot only. To help speed up the production of bile and detoxify your body.

6 **The gall bladder** **23**
Right foot only. To help release any tension in that part of your digestive system.

7 **The ileocaecal valve** **35**
Right foot only. To help prevent backflow of matter from your large to your small intestines.

8 **The sciatic nerve** **41**
To help release tension blocking the area.

9 **The hip and knee** **48**
To help reduce tension in these areas.

For a complete guide to the numbered points refer to the easy reference charts on pp 115-119

COMPLAINT:
Difficulty in releasing your bowel movements. You may expel a lot of gas. You may also get a sore anus and piles from straining the area.

CAUSE:
A general lack of vitality, weakness as a result of illness, holding on to emotional tensions or problems, stress, fear or lack of dietary fibre can all cause constipation. Not drinking enough water is a common factor. Irritable bowel syndrome (IBS), where the colon sometimes goes into spasm, infection, and allergies (particularly wheat and dairy) can also be problematic.

HOW REFLEXOLOGY HELPS:
Reflexology boosts your energy levels, frees up energy, helps to release blockages in your digestive system and helps your body to let go of stress and tension.

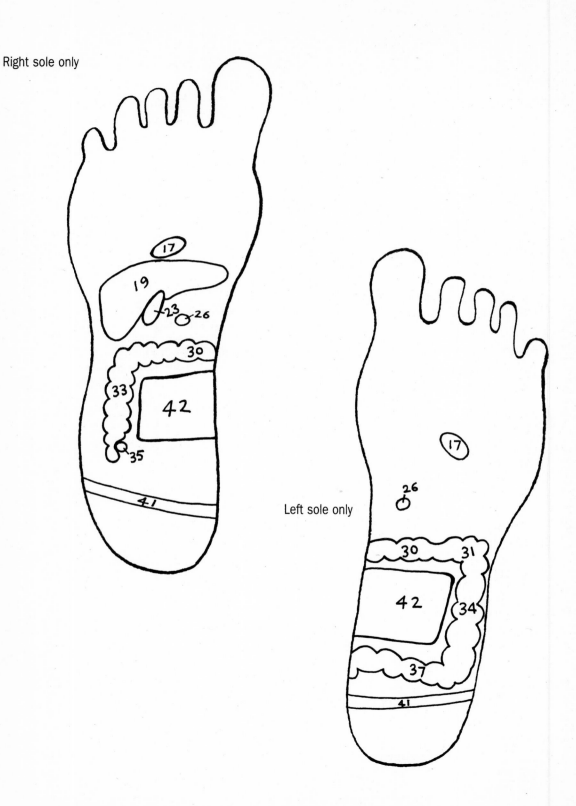

Right sole only

Left sole only

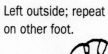

Left outside; repeat on other foot.

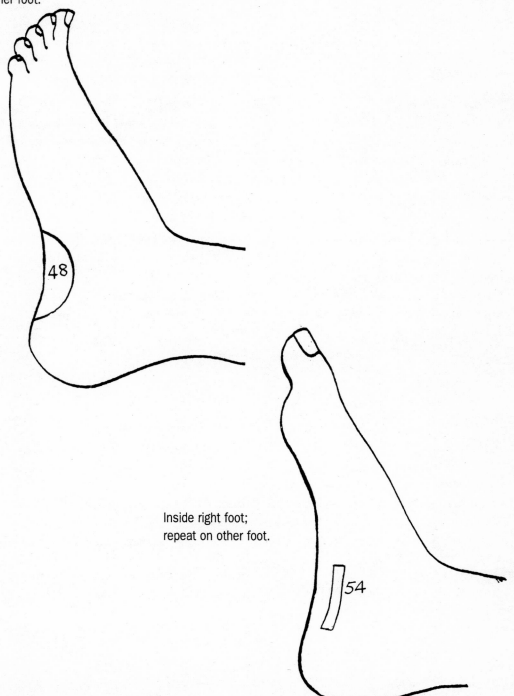

48

Inside right foot; repeat on other foot.

54

Diarrhoea

 TIME: 10 minutes, twice per day, on your hands. Practise the general relaxation techniques on pp 28-29 before and after this workout.

Work the following reflex areas on both hands except liver **19**, ileocaecal valve **35**, duodenum **24**, right hand only; anus **60**, left hand only.

1 The solar plexus 17
To help calm your nerves.

2 The ileocaecal valve 35
Right hand only. To help prevent the backflow of matter from your large to your small intestines.

3 The intestines 30, 31, 33, 34, 37, 42
To help balance the area.

4 The adrenal glands 26
To help balance your mineral levels. Hydrocortisone produced here can help you to fight any inflammation.

5 The duodenum 24
Right hand only. To help relax the area.

6 The liver 19
Right hand only. To help balance the output of bile and clear toxins from your body.

7 The anus 60
Left hand only. To help reduce discomfort.

8 The spine 52, 53, 54, 56
To help relax and calm your whole body.

9. The sacro-ileac joint 55
To help relax the lower back.

For a complete guide to the numbered points refer to the easy reference charts on pp 115-119

COMPLAINT:
Involuntary bowel movements which either are softer than usual or completely runny and non-stop, possibly resulting in you developing dehydration, a sore anus and a headache.

CAUSE:
You may get diarrhoea from food poisoning, allergies, shock or viral or bacterial infections. Fear or nervousness may also be a trigger for some people.

HOW REFLEXOLOGY HELPS:
Reflexology can help eliminate toxins, balance your mineral levels and calm you down. It is best to practise your self-help routine as soon as you get ill, either sitting or lying down.

Left top; repeat on
other hand.

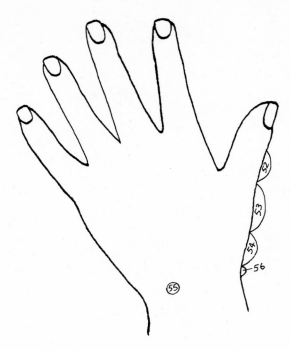

Left palm; repeat on other
hand except anus **60** .

Right palm only.

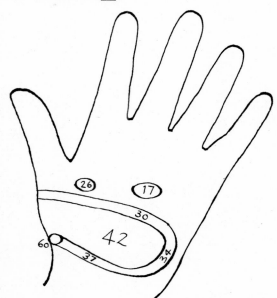

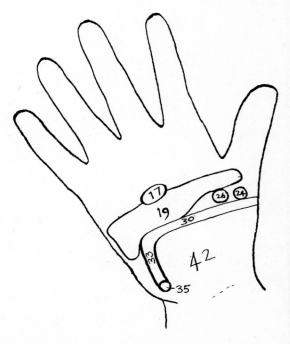

Panic Attack

 TIME: 5-10 minutes, at the onset of an attack, on your hands. Practise the general relaxation techniques on pp 28-29 before and after this workout.

Work the following reflex areas on both hands:

1 **The solar plexus** 17
   To help relax your nervous system and generally calm your whole body.

2 **The chest and lung** 13, the heart and heart-related areas 16 and the diaphragm 18

To help open up the ribcage to allow more oxygen into the area to help steady your breathing.

3 **The adrenal glands** 26
   To balance your energy levels.

For a complete guide to the numbered points refer to the easy reference charts on pp 115-119

COMPLAINT:

A panic attack makes you feel breathless, shivery and dizzy, and you may perspire.

CAUSES:

Panic attacks are caused by hyperventilation and can be triggered off by shock, stress or fear. Panic usually starts when you feel overwhelmed by a situation, a feeling of being out of control or being trapped. Agrophobics (who are scared of going out into open spaces) may have a panic attack when they leave home. You may have an attack if you are under pressure at work or at home or when you fear facing the unknown. You may also wake up in the middle of the night with a panic attack. At night fears which have been suppressed during the day often rise to the surface.

HOW REFLEXOLOGY HELPS:

Reflexology helps calm you down. You may also like to question yourself about the situation or problem in your life that is creating panic. Sit down with your two feet on the ground and your back straight when you practise these self-help movements.

Left palm only.

16

16

Right palm; repaet on other hand
except heart and heart-related
areas 16 .

13

17

18

18

16

26

Osteoporosis

 TIME: 15 minutes, twice per week, on your hands. Practise the general relaxation techniques on pp 28-29 before and after this workout.

Work the following reflex areas on both hands:

1 The pituitary `5`
To help you balance all the hormones in your body.

2 The thyroid and parathyroid `12`
To help balance the amount of calcium in your bones.

3 The ovaries `44`
To help release the hormone oestrogen directly into your bloodstream.

4 The spine `52`, `53`, `54`, `56`
To help increase your blood circulation, which carries the hormones around your body, and balance your whole nervous system.

5. The sacro-ileac joint `55`
To help relax the lower back.

For a complete guide to the numbered points refer to the easy reference charts on pp 115-119

COMPLAINT:
The bones in your body become thin and porous which can cause them to fracture and break easily.

CAUSE:
Osteoporosis is caused by a lack of female hormones, and/or nutrients important for bone strength such as calcium. You are more likely to get it during pregnancy, when you need a higher calcium intake or when the body's hormonal system may go out of balance easily, and after the menopause, as a result of lower levels of female hormones in your body.

HOW REFLEXOLOGY HELPS:
Reflexology helps increase your energy levels, boost your circulation and balance your hormone levels. It also helps the process of nutrient digestion into your body to keep your bones strong. If you are flexible then you may like to lie down and do this workout on your feet, otherwise sit down and practise on your hands. Remember to work gently using a very light pressure on your reflex points.

Left top; repeat
on other hand.

52

53

54

56

55

44

Left palm; repeat on
other hand

5

12

PART 4

Reference Section

List of Reflex Points on the Hands and Feet

1 TOP OF HEAD/BRAIN
2 TEETH AND SINUSES
3 TEMPORAL AREA
4 PINEAL/HYPOTHALAMUS
5 PITUITARY GLAND
6 BASE OF SKULL
7 SIDE OF NECK/LYMPH
8 NECK/THROAT
9 EYES
10 EARS
11 EUSTACHIAN TUBE
12 THYROID/PARATHYROID
13 CHEST/LUNGS
14 BRONCHIAL TUBES
15 ARMS/SHOULDERS
16 HEART AND HEART RELATED AREAS
17 SOLAR PLEXUS
18 DIAPHRAGM

19 LIVER
20 OESOPHAGUS
21 PYLORIC SPHINCTER
22 STOMACH
23 GALL BLADDER
24 DUODENUM
25 PANCREAS
26 ADRENALS
27 KIDNEYS
28 SPLEEN
29 HEPATIC FLECTURE
30 TRANSVERSE COLON
31 SPLENIC FLECTURE
32 URETER TUBES
33 ASCENDING COLON
34 DESCENDING COLON
35 ILEOCAECAL VALVE
36 BLADDER
37 SIGMOID COLON
38 CAECUM
39 APPENDIX
40 RECTUM

41 SCIATIC NERVE
42 SMALL INTESTINES
43 JAW/GUMS/TEETH
44 OVARIES/TESTES
45 UTERUS/PROSTATE
46 FALLOPIAN TUBES/
   SEMINAL VESICLES
47 BREAST
48 HIP/KNEE
49 LYMPHATICS
50 THYMUS
51 NOSE
52 CERVICAL SPINE
53 THORACIC SPINE
54 LUMBER SPINE
55 SACRO-ILEAC
56 COCCYX
57 UPPER LYMPH NODES/
   LYMPH BREAST
58 LYMPH GROIN
59 FACE
60 ANUS

SOLES OF THE FEET

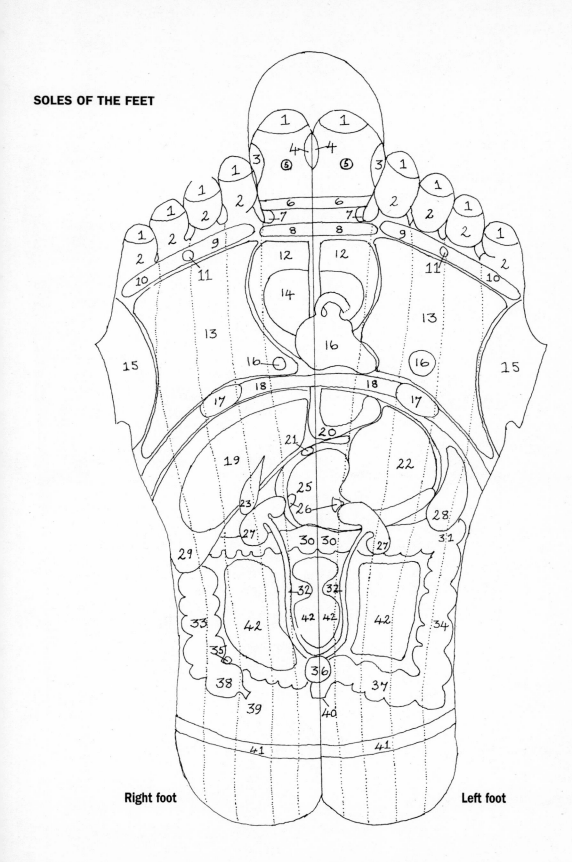

Right foot

Left foot

INSIDES OF THE FEET

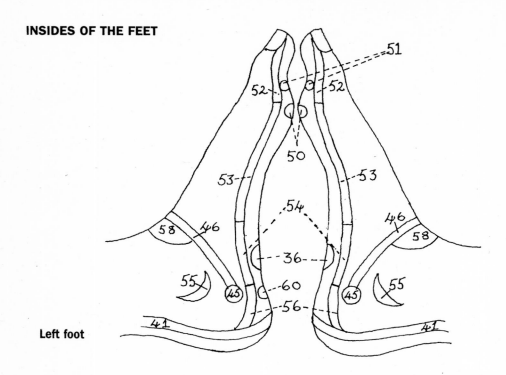

51

52 — 52

50

53 — — 53

54

58 46   46 58

36

55   55

45 — 60 45

— 56

41   41

Left foot   Right foot

OUTSIDES OF THE FEET

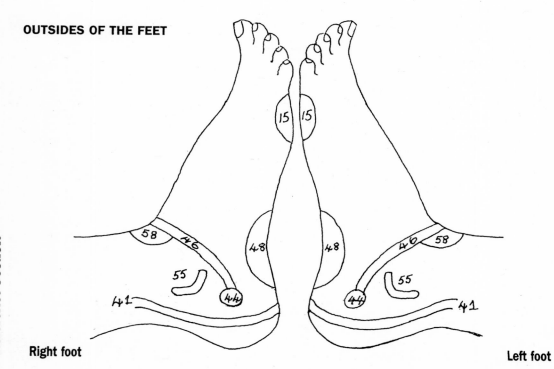

15 15

58 46   46 58

48 48

55   55

44   44

41   41

Right foot   Left foot

TOPS OF THE FEET

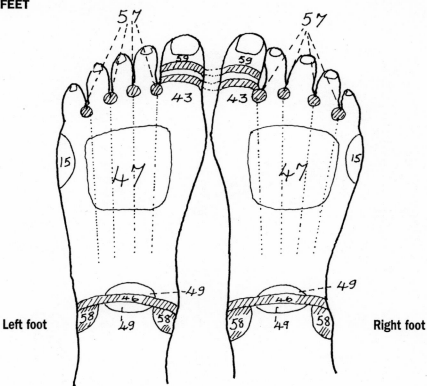

Left foot   Right foot

List of Reflex Points on the Hands and Feet

1 TOP OF HEAD/BRAIN	19 LIVER	41 SCIATIC NERVE
2 TEETH AND SINUSES	20 OESOPHAGUS	42 SMALL INTESTINES
3 TEMPORAL AREA	21 PYLORIC SPHINCTER	43 JAW/GUMS/TEETH
4 PINEAL/HYPOTHALAMUS	22 STOMACH	44 OVARIES/TESTES
5 PITUITARY GLAND	23 GALL BLADDER	45 UTERUS/PROSTATE
6 BASE OF SKULL	24 DUODENUM	46 FALLOPIAN TUBES/
7 SIDE OF NECK/LYMPH	25 PANCREAS	SEMINAL VESICLES
8 NECK/THROAT	26 ADRENALS	47 BREAST
9 EYES	27 KIDNEYS	48 HIP/KNEE
10 EARS	28 SPLEEN	49 LYMPHATICS
11 EUSTACHIAN TUBE	29 HEPATIC FLECTURE	50 THYMUS
12 THYROID/PARATHYROID	30 TRANSVERSE COLON	51 NOSE
13 CHEST/LUNGS	31 SPLENIC FLECTURE	52 CERVICAL SPINE
14 BRONCHIAL TUBES	32 URETER TUBES	53 THORACIC SPINE
15 ARMS/SHOULDERS	33 ASCENDING COLON	54 LUMBER SPINE
16 HEART AND HEART RELATED AREAS	34 DESCENDING COLON	55 SACRO-ILEAC
17 SOLAR PLEXUS	35 ILEOCAECAL VALVE	56 COCCYX
18 DIAPHRAGM	36 BLADDER	57 UPPER LYMPH NODES/
	37 SIGMOID COLON	LYMPH BREAST
	38 CAECUM	58 LYMPH GROIN
	39 APPENDIX	59 FACE
	40 RECTUM	60 ANUS

Reference Section

PALMS OF THE HANDS

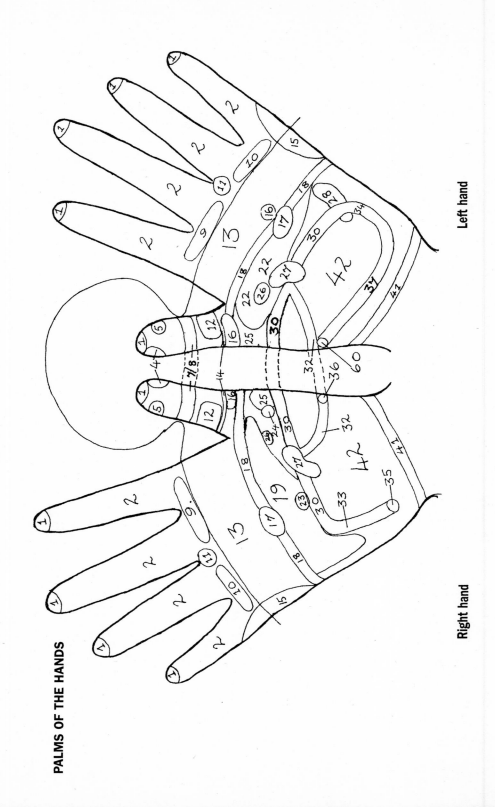

Left hand

Right hand

TOPS OF THE HANDS

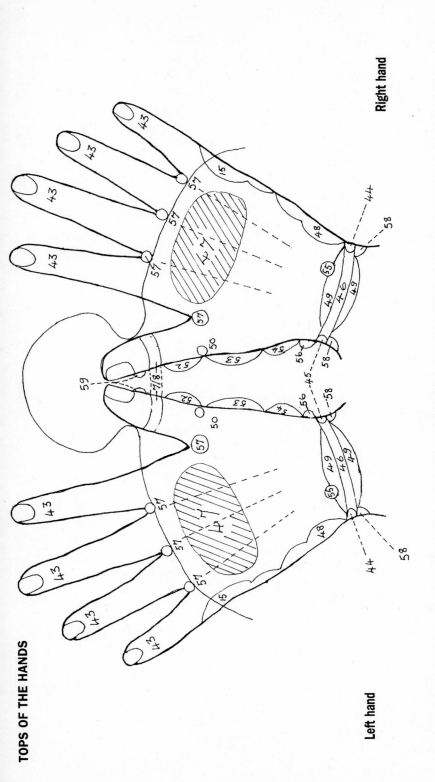

Left hand

Right hand

List of Reflex Points on the Hands and Feet

1 TOP OF HEAD/BRAIN
2 TEETH AND SINUSES
3 TEMPORAL AREA
4 PINEAL/HYPOTHALAMUS
5 PITUITARY GLAND
6 BASE OF SKULL
7 SIDE OF NECK/LYMPH
8 NECK/THROAT
9 EYES
10 EARS

11 EUSTACHIAN TUBE
12 THYROID/PARATHYROID
13 CHEST/LUNGS
14 BRONCHIAL TUBES
15 ARMS/SHOULDERS
16 HEART AND HEART RELATED
   AREAS
17 SOLAR PLEXUS
18 DIAPHRAGM
19 LIVER
20 OESOPHAGUS
21 PYLORIC SPHINCTER
22 STOMACH
23 GALL BLADDER

24 DUODENUM
25 PANCREAS
26 ADRENALS
27 KIDNEYS
28 SPLEEN
29 HEPATIC FLECTURE
30 TRANSVERSE COLON
31 SPLENIC FLECTURE
32 URETER TUBES
33 ASCENDING COLON
34 DESCENDING COLON
35 ILEOCAECAL VALVE
36 BLADDER
37 SIGMOID COLON

38 CAECUM
39 APPENDIX
40 RECTUM
41 SCIATIC NERVE
42 SMALL INTESTINES
43 JAW/GUMS/TEETH
44 OVARIES/TESTES
45 UTERUS/PROSTATE
46 FALLOPIAN TUBES/SEMINAL
   VESICLES
47 BREAST
48 HIP/KNEE
49 LYMPHATICS
50 THYMUS

51 NOSE
52 CERVICAL SPINE
53 THORACIC SPINE
54 LUMBER SPINE
55 SACRO-ILEAC
56 COCCYX
57 UPPER LYMPH NODES/ LYMPH
   BREAST
58 LYMPH GROIN
59 FACE
60 ANUS

Easy Reference Charts

Visiting a Professional Reflexologist

Visiting a professional reflexologist is very different from working on your own hands and feet because the reflexologist is experienced to detect the whole picture of your health and can be objective. Being totally objective about your own health is almost impossible because you know yourself and cannot be detached from your symptoms. The reflexologist gives you the full care and attention you deserve during your visit, which usually lasts a full hour. You may think it is indulgent to set aside time for yourself for reflexology, especially if you lead an hectic lifestyle or have always been caring for others. But it is essential to allow yourself this time, even if you are healthy, so that you can relax and let go of worries, and enjoy being pampered.

Like all complementary (or alternative) therapies, reflexology offers you the chance to look at the cause and the behavioural patterns attributed to your health problems. For instance, if you are always seeking approval you may find out why you are stuck in this pattern and try to change it if you choose. This is different from conventional medicine, which treats symptoms as the problem.

Reflexologists do not claim to cure you, treat a specific illness or prescribe any medicines for you (only doctors are allowed to do this), but reflexology helps bring balance to your mind, body and spirit by addressing the cause of your problems through relaxation and the stimulation of your body's natural healing powers. As already mentioned, reflexology encourages you to take responsibility for your own health and your own life and encourages self-awareness.

When Should You Visit a Reflexologist?

You can visit a reflexologist for pure pleasure – to enjoy the luxury of your feet being 'massaged' for an hour! This can help to keep you happy, relaxed and in optimum health. However you are more likely to visit a reflexologist when you are already ill, run down or stressed; when your body has gone out of balance. In some cases, people will say that they are too ill to visit a reflexologist, but a session during most illnesses can be extremely beneficial.

Preparing for a Reflexology Treatment

If your feet don't smell 'pretty' at the end of the day then you can appreciate that washing your feet or hands before a reflexology treatment is kind to your reflexologist. Also, avoid a heavy meal, otherwise your body will be working overtime and may not be able to relax fully and enjoy the maximum benefits of the treatment.

The Initial Reflexology Consultation

Your first visit to a reflexologist may last longer than a normal session because you'll need to give your basic medical history (even if you are healthy) and discuss your lifestyle. This includes any past or present medication, operations and emotional upsets or traumas experienced in your life, but any information you give is confidential. If you are taking medication, have had a recent operation or significant illness you will be required to give your reflexologist a doctor's 'permission note' from your GP or consultant. In this way the reflexologist can work in cooperation with your doctor to help keep you healthy and in your best interests.

From the information on your consultation form and after your first treatment, the reflexologist can give you an indication as to how many more treatments you will need and when to visit. Once or twice a week is usual, but it may be more or less, according to your problem. It is very difficult to tell exactly how long you'll need treatment because everyone reacts differently. It is very common for people to continue with treatment long after their problem has disappeared because they enjoy reflexology so much and look forward to setting aside time for themselves regularly.

Occasionally, at the initial consultation any good reflexologist may recommend some other form of complementary therapy other than reflexology for you if they believe it would suit you better, for example, osteopathy, acupuncture, massage, shiatsu, cranial sacral therapy, etc. Many people experiment with different therapies to see which one they prefer; this is fine but it is best to stay with one therapy over a period of time.

On your first visit to a reflexologist you may feel fearful or nervous because you don't know what to expect and you may not know your reflexologist. You may feel embarrassed about your problem or even by the state of your feet! This is completely normal. Your reflexologist will help to make you feel comfortable, so that you can get the most out of your treatments.

After your written consultation you lie or sit down and take off your shoes, tights or socks (loose clothing or trousers offer the most comfort). The reflexologist first uses an antiseptic wipe on your feet or hands, and then applies talc (usually unperfumed and aluminium free), an aqueous cream or base oil. You may be asked to take some deep breaths; relax and know that you are in the safe, caring hands of a professional.

How Much Does It Cost?

Reflexologists all charge different fees, so always remember to check the price of a treatment before you book your appointment. Many reflexologists offer concessions for the unemployed or senior citizens, or discounts for booking a course (which is normally paid for in full before it begins).

During a Reflexology Session

Sometimes you may want to talk whilst receiving reflexology and other times you'll like to be quiet; the reflexologist will be happy to listen to your problems.

The general relaxation techniques are applied first to work your whole body and then the reflexologist concentrates on any problem areas detected in your hands or feet. Toxins or problems areas are worked on to release the congestion to help the body find its own equilibrium. If you are healthy and receiving reflexology as a treat or to help with preventative healthcare, the reflexologist will still give you a complete treatment.

How Will I React During a Session?

Reactions vary at each session and with each treatment, and are different for everyone. You may feel very energetic and light, as though all your problems have floated away, you may feel tired and your body heavy, you may be emotional or even fall asleep. Sometimes when you enter a deep state of relaxation you may suddenly feel cold or shivery. You may feel tingling in your hands or feet or all through your body as the reflexology releases blockages that enables any stagnant energies to flow freely.

A reason why you may become emotional during a session is because each reflex point carries with it memories and pressing certain points can cause you to release these memories. For example, if you had been holding on to anger or resentment towards someone, whether from childhood or from a recent situation, in one part of your body, then when the reflexologist presses that reflex area a memory is released. You may suddenly get angry or burst into tears and remember the incident vividly. This is completely normal and you may choose to talk about it with your therapist. It is an essential part of the healing process and helps your body to clear away anything that is blocking and preventing it from healing itself, physically, emotionally or mentally.

Will Reflexology Hurt?

This depends upon your condition. If you are generally very healthy but have a blocked sinus from a cold, for example, then these reflex points may be painful temporarily. If you have a specific illness which you have been suffering from for many years then the corresponding reflex points may feel very tender or sore. However, sometimes you may not feel any pain during your first few visits because the problem is 'buried' deep in your body. As the sessions progress you may gradually feel sensation in these points, which is the illness or problem releasing. Eventually the pain diminishes as the symptoms improve and balance out. It is also possible that a completely healthy person may feel sensitivity and the reflexologist will work carefully when a sensitive part is found.

Pain and sensitivity are indicators that your body is out of balance or ill. You can help yourself by asking, 'Why have I got this illness/problem? What can I do about it? How can reflexology help me with it?' Ignoring persistent pain is dangerous because it may turn into a chronic or acute problem later on. Learn to listen to your body and the messages it's giving you.

After a Reflexology Session

You may feel tired and sleep very well after receiving reflexology or you may be very energetic; reflexology both relaxes and stimulates your body. Some people also experience feelings of anger or sadness, or may be weepy – this is completely normal and it is best to let out any emotions rather than suppress them.

Immediately after your treatment your urine will usually be darker in colour as toxins are released from your body. You may occasionally find yourself perspiring more or you may develop a skin rash over an area where there were a lot of toxins which have been released through the skin, and so on. So drink plenty of water after your treatment. It is best to have no expectations, as your body will react differently to each session.

To obtain the maximum benefits from your treatment it is best if you avoid any strenuous activities immediately afterwards and simply allow your body to relax.

Your symptoms may feel worse for a short time after your treatment, as they rise to the surface to be healed and clear through your body. It is also possible that after a number of treatments (it varies with everyone) your symptoms may become very intense and appear much worse than when you actually started your first session. You may feel a sense of hopelessness about your illness and think that the reflexology isn't working. But this usually means that it is working very well because it is clearing everything away to get to the root cause of your illness, whilst working on your whole body. You may consider stopping your treatments because you can't see any end to your problems. Try to stay with this process and work through it. In complementary therapy terms it is called a 'healing crisis' – everything comes to a head.

You may experience a little healing crisis or, if you have been ill for many years and there are deep problems being faced, you may experience an intense one. Like all cycles in life, nothing ever stays the same and change occurs daily. No day is ever exactly the same as the next day and the same cycles can be applied to your illness. So no one can say how long your crisis may last – a day, a month or a year or more – but sooner or later it will move on.

Sometimes people may switch to another complementary therapy at this time, believing it will help more. Whatever course of action you decide to take it is fine and the reflexologist can take no responsibility for the decisions you make in your life or the effects the treatment is having upon your body, because you are choosing that experience. And at the time of your healing crisis you need to take extra care and responsibility for yourself.

How Do I Find a Professional Reflexologist in my Area?

Look at the list of professional associations on page 124, or ask at your local surgery or health centre. Many reflexologists work from home and sometimes may call at your home.

PROFESSIONAL CONTACTS

For details of professional reflexologists in your area, or for professional training, contact:

The Association of Reflexologists
27 Old Gloucester Street
London WC1 3XX
UK

The British Reflexology Association
12 Pond Road
London SE3 6JL
UK

CIRL
Via Bronzino 11
20133 Milan
Italy

Deutscher Reflexologen Verband
Helga Dittman
Lloyd G. Wells Street
14163 Berlin
Germany

Forend Danske Zone Terapeuter
Chr. Winthersvej 13
6000 Kolding
Denmark

The Reflexology Association of America
4012 South Rainbow Bvd
Box K585
Las Vegas
NV89 1032059
USA

The Reflexology Association of Australia
PO Box 841
Narradeen
NSW 2101
Australia

The South African Reflexology Society
Box 201858
Durban North 4016
Republic of South Africa

FURTHER READING

Brennan, Barbara Ann, *Hands of Light*, Bantam New Age Books, USA, 1988
This book is a wonderful guide to the rudiments of healing and also offers deeper insights into life. It shows a good understanding of personality and psychological patterns. The title is very apt, as a result of the beautiful illustrations.

You may also like to explore Barbara Brennan's second book, *Light Emerging*, 1994, which offers an in-depth adventure into all areas of healing. It also gives examples of the way you use your energy, both positive and negative, in everyday life, and how it affects others.

Dougans, Inge, with Ellis, Suzanne, *The Art of Reflexology*, Element Books, 1992
This very well researched book presents an excellent view of how reflexology works with the Chinese meridian system. Reflexology traditionally recognizes the 10 vertical zones or energy pathways as the way energies flow through the body, but this book has adapted the Chinese meridians to work with the overall treatment when practising reflexology. There is also a section on the Five Elements - earth, fire, metal, wood and water - explaining their relevance to health and reflexology.

Gillanders, Ann, *Step by Step Guide to Reflexology*, Gaia Books, 1995
This book is a clearly illustrated and easy to follow guide to reflexology, with something for beginners right through to adepts. Its design is uplifting and it is warm and open and really welcomes you in to try some of these wonderful techniques.

Ingham, Eunice, *Stories the Feet Can Tell*, Ingham Publications, USA, 1992
Reflexology to uplift and inspire you from one of its pioneers.

Norman, Laura, with Cowan, Thomas, *The Reflexology Handbook*, Piatkus, 1988
This is an excellent, straightforward and easy to understand reflexology book which is very concise and practical. It covers many subjects, ranging from reflexology for children to reflexology and health care professionals, and also contains affirmations to enhance positive thinking

Stormer, Chris, *Language of the Feet*, Headway, 1995
This book focuses on reading your feet – colour, shape, temperature, positioning of corns and blisters etc., even toe-nail reading - in order to give information to the reflexologist in conjunction with the treatment. Non-professionals will also find this well illustrated book absolutely fascinating!

There are so many excellent books available on reflexology at my bookstore, each offering its own unique approach to the subject, that is has been difficult to single out these few. So remember to allow yourself plenty of time to browse around your local bookshop to find the right book for you. Have fun!

BIOGRAPHY

SONIA DUCIE
Member of the Association of
Reflexologists

Sonia Ducie studied the Eunice Ingham
method of reflexology in 1990 with
Margaret Bonner-Walter in London and
has been practising reflexology for over
six years in clinics and in private practice.
Sonia teaches self-help reflexology at
workshops in London. She is also a
professional numerologist.

CHARLES JAMES HORAN
Member of the Association of
Reflexologists

Jim Horan has been practising reflexology
for over eight years and trained with the
Gaia School of Reflexology in Shropshire,
using the Doreen Bayley method. Jim has
been very active in promoting reflexology
and teaching at workshops and colleges.
He has researched and designed maps of
the hands and feet as illustrated in this
book. Jim also practises Bio-Mobility -
body alignment through the manipulation
of muscles.

INDEX

Index